PHARMACEUTICAL ENGINEERING
Experimental Lab Manual - I (UNIT OPERATIONS)

Dr.Jayapal Reddy Gangadi
M.Pharm, FICCP, Ph.D
Associate Professor,
(Editor-in-Chief, IJPBS)
Talla Padmavathi Pharmacy College
Warangal, Telangana State
India

Copyright

All rights reserved. No part of this book may be reproduced or transmitted in any form or by any means, electronic or mechanical including photocopying, recording, or any information storage and retrieval system without the prior written permission from the publisher and the copyright holder.

Copyright © 2017-Dr. Jayapal Reddy Gangadi

All rights reserved.

ISBN-13: 978-1545236642

ISBN-10: 154523664X

Dedication

This book is dedicated to

My family members and Teachers

Foreword

Prof. J.Venkateshwar Rao
M.Pharm, Ph.D
Principal, Talla Padmavathi College of Pharmacy
Warangal, India.

I am very much happy to express myself about this book and author. This book consists of 17 experiments and each experiment consists of theory part as well as experimental procedures. All experiments were explained diagrammatically (all diagrams in this book designed by author with the help of Edraw Max software). This book is simple and easy to understand for the teachers as well as students. This book also contains definitions and Viva-Voce questions for each topic.

Regarding author, he graduated from our college only and completed his post-graduation from Annamalai University, Chidambaram, Chennai. He completed his Ph.D from Acharya Nagarjuna University, Guntur, Andhra Pradesh, under my guidance.

Preface

This book has been written with an intention to cover all the possible experiments which are to be conducted in the pharmaceutical engineering/ Pharmaceutical Unit Operations laboratory at the UG level. I have tried to incorporate all the experiments suggested under pharmaceutical engineering / Pharmaceutical Unit Operations by various universities.

The designed experiments are all practically performed in the laboratory by my students and that has given me ample to chance to improve the quality of the experiments. During this period, I could observe the difficulties of the students in collecting primary information which are the part of the main experiments. That is the usage of different standard values like specific heat, radiation constants of different materials and conversion of units are examples. I have included all such information in this book so students are benefited to get them in a single book and also incorporated useful definitions, Viva Questions and related Questions to that individual experiments.

I am so proud to present before you my book *"Pharmaceutical Engineering Experimental Lab Manual-I (Unit Operations)"*. Hope that it will be well accepted by the Pharmaceutical science community.

The suggestions are encouraged and acknowledged.

-**Author**

Acknowledgements

The author express their heartfelt thanks to *Dr. J. Venkateshwar Rao*, Principal, Talla Padmavathi College of Pharmacy and *Dr. Sanjeev Kumar Subudhi*, Principal, Talla Padmavathi Pharmacy college, Warangal for their constant encouragement and help.

The author express their sincere thanks to *Sri.Talla Mallesham*, Chairman, LS Educational Society and *Mr. Talla Varun*, Academic director, Talla Padmavathi Pharmacy Colleges, Warangal for their affection and encouragement.

April 2017   **-Author**

Contents

Foreword

Preface

Acknowledgements

Symbols

SECTION I: FLOW OF FLUIDS

Expt-1: Determination of Reynold's Number and Frictional Factor By Calculating Frictional Losses. 01

Expt-2: Determination of Reynold's Number By Calculating Velocity of Fluids And Area Of Pipes 06

SECTION II: HEAT TRANSFER

Expt-3: Determination of Radiation Constant of Iron Cylinder 12

Expt-4: Determination of Radiation Constant of Brass Cylinder 25

Expt-5: Determination of Radiation Constant of Unpainted and Painted Glass 30

Expt-6: Determination of Overall Heat Transfer coefficients 39

SECTION-III: EVAPORATION

Expt-7: Determination of Factors Affecting Rate Of Evaporation 48

SECTION-IV: DISTILLATION

Expt-8: Preparation of Azeotropic Alcohol-Azeotropic Distillation 58

SECTION-V: DRYING

Expt-9: Determination of Rate of Drying, Free Moisture Content and Bound Moisture Content 67

SECTION-VI: FILTRATION

Expt-10: Effect of Factors on Filtration Rate-Materials Related Factors (Effect of Filter Aids on Rate of Filtration).................................77

Expt-11: Effect of Factors on Filtration Rate-Process Related Factors...82

SECTION-VII: HUMIDITY

Expt-12: Determination of Humidity-Psychometric Method..................88

Expt-13: Determination of Humidity-Dew Point Method......................96

SECTION-VIII: SIZE REDUCTION AND SEPARATION

Expt-14: Determination of Efficiency of Size Reduction of a Mixer and a Ball Mill..101

SECTION-IX: MIXING

Expt-15: Mixing Index of a Blender - Calcium Carbonate and Talc 109

SECTION X: CRYSTALLIZATION

Expt-16: Effect of Various Factors on The Nature of Crystal Growth of Supersaturated Solutions by Different Methods........................123

Expt-17: Determination of Crystallization By Shock Cooling...............127

DEFINITIONS..**135**

VIVA QUESTIONS..**154**

BIBLIOGRAPHY...**160**

Symbols

ρ	=	Density (lb mass / cu.ft.)
μ, η	=	Viscosity (lb mass / ft.sec)
β	=	Coefficient of thermal expansion; angle
π	=	constant (22/7 = 3.14)
α	=	Radiation constant
θ	=	Time (Sec)
Δ	=	Finite difference
λ	=	Latent heat of vaporization
g	=	Acceleration of gravity
r	=	Radius
d	=	Diameter
u	=	Average velocity
Re	=	Raynolds Number
f	=	Friction Factor
A	=	Area
s	=	Specific heat of metal cylinder
h	=	height of metal cylinder

Section I
Flow of Fluids

Expt-1: Determination of Reynold's Number and Frictional Factor by Calculating Frictional Losses.

AIM: To determine Reynold's Number and frictional factor by calculating frictional losses in pipes in which fluids are flowing.

REQUIREMENTS:

Tubes of pipes; Measuring cylinders (1000 ml); Vernier calipers and Beakers.

OBJECTIVES:

i. Passing of reactants (liquids or gases) into the reaction system.
ii. Transferring of air, nutrient broth into the fermenter.
iii. Bottling of liquid (dosage forms) medicaments into suitable containers.
iv. Transportation of sterile air and sterile water in the production of parenterals.

v. Mixing of solids and liquids in case of suspensions.

vi. Packing of semisolids in containers.

PRINCIPLE:

The term '*fluids*' include both liquids and gases. The flow of fluids through a closed channel is influenced by various factors. The flow can be either viscous or turbulent and this can be observed in classical Reynold's experiment. When a fluid is passing through a pipe of uniform diameter at very slow motion, one can observe a laminar flow. This is because, the fluid flow is parallel straight lines and this is also known as "Viscous or Streamline flow".

There are two forms of fluid motions, viscous flow and turbulent flow. The velocity at which the flow changes from one kind of flow to other is known as the "Critical Velocity". The critical velocity depends on diameter of tube, velocity of fluid, density of liquid, viscosity of liquid. By knowing Reynold's number, we can determine the type of flow, the liquid exhibit.

The factors, which affect the mechanism of fluid flow, are diameter, D, average velocity, u, density of liquid, ρ, and viscosity of the fluid, μ.

Reynold's number (R_e) can be calculated as:

$$R_e = Du\rho / \mu$$

Where,

> D = Diameter of pipe/ tube (m); u = Velocity of fluid (m/s); ρ = density of fluid (for water = 1 kg/m³); μ = viscosity of fluid (for water 0.01 poise or kg/ m.s).

Reynold's number is a dimensionless number. For straight circular pipes, the value of R_e is less than 2,100 and flow will always be viscous/ stream line. When value of R_e is over 4,000, the flow will always be turbulent. Between 2,100 and 4,000, a *transition region* is found where the flow may be either laminar or turbulent, depending upon conditions at the entrance of the tube and on the distance from the entrance.

Fictional Factor:

In the fluid flowing through a circular pipe of length, the total force resisting the flow must equal the product divided by the cross-sectional area of the pipe, since pressure is measured in force per unit area. This can be represented in terms of Reynold's number and frictional factor.

$$f = 16/R_e$$

PROCEDURE:

1. Take a jar, and fill the jar with one liter of water, and mark the upper level of the water with the permanent marker.
2. Now, select different types of pipes, and measure their diameter.

3. Then, connect one end of the pipes to reservoir of water such that, the velocity of the flowing through pipe can be varied. Three different pipes of varying diameter are connected to three different taps.
4. From each pipe collect water (one liter) each time by varying speeds (Low, Medium and High). Time taken for the collection of water in each case is noted.
5. Calculate the velocity of water.
6. From the readings taken, Re and frictional factor are calculated.
7. Plot a graph between Re and Frictional factor (*f*).

OBSERVATIONS AND CALCULATIONS:

Reynold's Number, $R_e = Du\rho / \mu$

Frictional factor can be calculated by using formula $(f) = 16/R_e$

Table 1.1:

Pipes	Diameter of pipe (D)	Radius of pipe (r)	Area (A) πr^2	Time taken to collect 1000 ml water	Avg. Velocity= Volume/Area x time	$R_e = Du\rho / \mu$	$f = 16/R_e$

Graph:

Graph between Re (X-axis) and Frictional factor (*f*) (Y-axis).

REPORT:

From the observation made, it is inferred that, as velocity of flow of fluid increases, Reynold's number increases while the frictional factor decreases. With increase in diameter of the pipe, Reynold's number increases.

Reynolds number was found to be =_____

Expt-2: Determination of Reynold's Number by Calculating Velocity of Fluids and Area of Pipes

AIM:

To determine the Reynold's number by calculating velocity of fluids and Area of pipes in which fluids are flowing.

Requirements:

Tubes of pipes; Measuring cylinders (1000 ml); Vernier calipers and Beakers.

OBJECTIVES:

i. Passing of reactants (liquids or gases) into the reaction system.
ii. Transferring of air, nutrient broth into the fermenter.
iii. Bottling of liquid (dosage forms) medicaments into suitable containers.
iv. Transportation of sterile air and sterile water in the production of parenterals.
v. Mixing of solids and liquids in case of suspensions.
vi. Packing of semisolids in containers.

Section-I   Expt-2: Reynolds Number-Velocity and Area

PRINCIPLE:

The term '*fluids*' include both liquids and gases. The flow of fluids through a closed channel is influenced by various factors. The flow can be either viscous or turbulent and this can be observed in classical Reynold's experiment. When a fluid is passing through a pipe of uniform diameter at very slow motion, one can observe a laminar flow. This is because, the fluid flow is parallel straight lines and this is also known as "**Viscous or Streamline flow**".

There are two forms of fluid motions, **viscous flow, and turbulent flow**. The velocity at which the flow changes from one kind of flow to other is known as the "**Critical Velocity**". The critical velocity depends on diameter of tube, velocity of fluid, density of liquid, viscosity of liquid. By knowing Reynold's number, we can determine the type of flow, the liquid exhibit.

The factors, which affect the mechanism of fluid flow, are diameter, D, average velocity, u, density of liquid, ρ, and viscosity of the fluid, μ.

Reynold's number (R_e) can be calculated as:

$$R_e = Du\rho / \mu$$

Where,

D= Diameter of pipe/ tube (m); u=Velocity of fluid (m/s); ρ=density of fluid (for water = 1 kg/m^3); μ= viscosity of fluid (for water 0.01 poise or kg/ m.s).

Reynold's number is a dimensionless number. For straight circular pipes, the value of R_e is less than 2,100 and flow will always be viscous/ stream line. When value of R_e is over 4,000, the flow will always be turbulent. Between 2,100 and 4,000, a *transition region* is found where the flow may be either laminar or turbulent, depending upon conditions at the entrance of the tube and on the distance from the entrance.

Significance of Reynold's number:

- It can be used to predict the nature (Viscous or Turbulent) of flow in a particular set of circumstances.
- The physical stability of suspension depends on the rate of settling of the particles.
- Rate of sedimentation of particles must not be too rapid to create turbulence. Stoke's Law is modified to include Reynold's number. Therefore, the type of flow (whether laminar or turbulent) is important.
- The rate of heat transfer in liquids also depends on the flow, whether viscous or turbulent, etc.

PROCEDURE:

1. Collect the two water reservoirs, one for colour water and another one, normal water.
2. Get a pipe line/ tube line, which is transparent and should be connected one end to the coloured water reservoir, and normal

water reservoir connected in between pipe line as shown in diagram.
3. In Reynold's experiment, a glass tube is connected to a reservoir of water in such a way that the capacity of water flowing through the tube could be varied at wall.
4. In the inlet end of the tube a nozzle is inserted through which a fine stream of coloured water could be introduced.

CONCLUSION:

Reynold's found that when the velocity of the water was low, thread of colour maintained itself throughout the tube. By putting in more than one of these jets at different points in cross section, it can be shown that in no part of the tube was there any mixing, and the fluid flowed in parallel, straight lines.

OBSERVATION AND CALCULATIONS:

Reynold's Number, $R_e = D u \rho / \mu$

Table 2.1:

Pipes	Diameter of pipe (D)	Radius of pipe (r)	Area (A) πr^2	Time taken to collect 1000 ml water	Avg. Velocity= Volume/Area x time	$R_e = D u \rho / \mu$	$f = 16/R_e$

Pharmaceutical Engineering Experimental Lab Manual-I (Unit Operations)

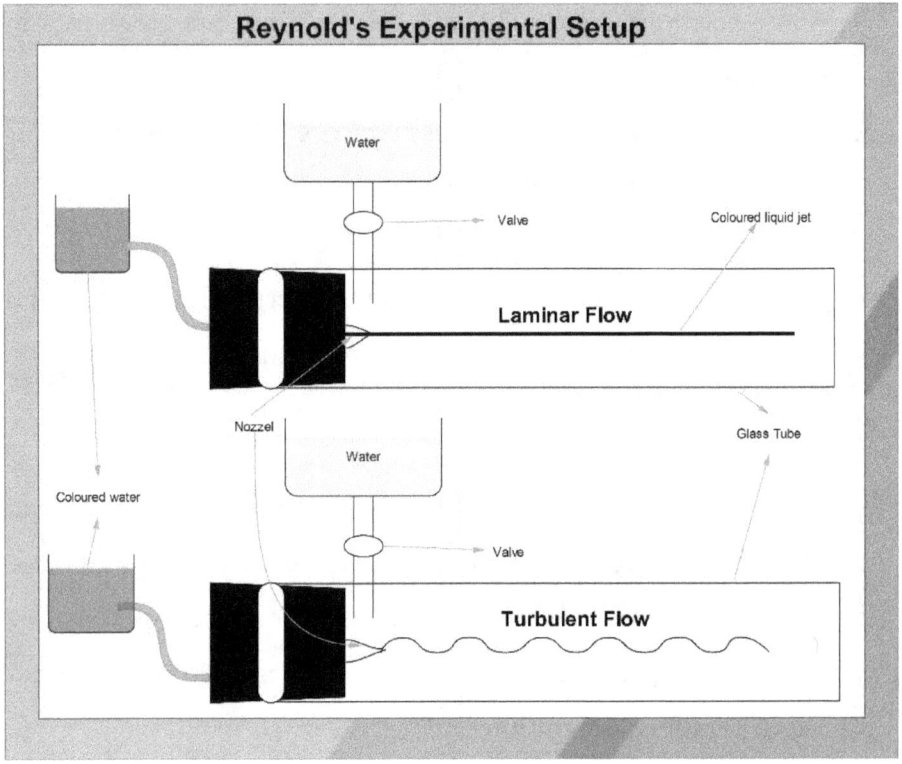

REPORT:

Reynold's Number was found to be= _____

QUESTIONS:

1. Why do we use Reynolds number?
2. Compare the results obtained through calculations and observations. State whether or not the results are reasonable. If not, explain the reasons?
3. Is the Reynolds number obtained dependent on tube size or shape?

4. Draw a fully developed laminar and turbulent velocity profile (pipe flow). Explain why they are different.
5. How is Reynolds number designed for:
   a) Flow in a circular pipe of diameter, D?
   b) Flow in a rectangular duct of cross section a x b?

Osborne Reynolds

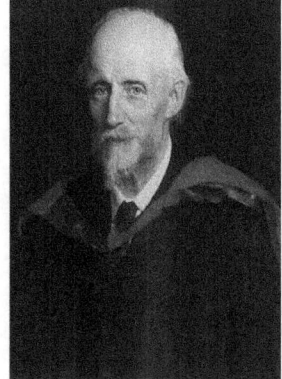

A British engineer to first observe and classify different types of flow.

Reynolds most famously studied the conditions in which the flow of fluid in pipes transitioned from laminar flow to turbulent flow. In 1883 Reynolds demonstrated the transition to turbulent flow in a classic experiment in which he examined the behaviour of water flow under different flow rates using a small jet of dyed water introduced into the centre of flow in a larger pipe.

@@@♥♥@@@

SECTION II
HEAT TRANSFER

Expt-3: Determination of Radiation Constant of Iron Cylinder

AIM: To determine Radiation constant of Iron cylinder and to interpret influence of temperature on Radiation Constant.

APPARATUS REQUIRED:

Iron cylinder, Tripod stand, Thermometer, Wooden plank and Stop clock.

THEORY:

Heat Transfer is a major unit operation. Heat flows from a region of high temperature to a region of low temperature. Understanding of heat transfer requires study of the mechanisms and rate of process. Heat may flow by one or more of the 3 basic mechanisms:

i. Conduction: is a process in which heat flow in a body is achieved by the transfer of the momentum of the individual atoms or molecules without mixing. Example: flow of heat through the metal shell of a boiler takes place by conduction as far as solid shell or wall is considered. This mechanism is limited to solids and fluids.

ii. Convection: is a process in which heat flow is achieved by actual mixing of warmer portions with cooler portions of the same materials. Example: heating of water by a hot surface (coil type water heater) is mainly by convection. Convection currents are responsible for winds, land and sea breezes, ocean currents etc.

iii. Radiation: is a process in which heat flows through spaces by means of electromagnetic waves. Example: a black surface absorbs most of the radiation received by it.

Thermal Radiation: Heat transfer by radiation is known as *thermal radiation*. All solid bodies radiate energy, when their temperatures are above absolute zero.

Applications: Radiation (thermal) energy is used in different processes, where heat is necessary. For example, drying of solids is attempted using micro-wave radiation, IR radiation etc.

PRINCIPLE:

A freely suspended hot body looses heat by conduction, convection, and radiation, until it reaches the room temperature. This is an equilibrium condition. In this system, the heat loss through convection is neglected, since movement of particles is negligible. As the metal cylinder is freely suspended without any contact with the metal the heat loss through conduction is considered minimum.

For this reason, the metal cylinder is placed on a glass tripod stand (Figure).

It two adjacent surfaces are at different temperature; the hotter body radiates more than it receives and its temperature falls. The cooler surface receives more energy than it emits and its temperature rises. Ultimately, thermal equilibrium is reached.

Stefan-Boltzmann law gives the total amount of radiation emitted by a body:

$$q = bAT^4 \quad \ldots\ldots\ldots(01)$$

Where, q = energy radiated per second, W or J/s; A = Area of radiating surface, m²; T = Absolute temperature of the radiating surface, K; b = Constant, W/m². K⁴

The above equation (01), the rate of heating depends upon the temperature and surface area of the emitter and the absorption capacity of the material to be heated.

The difference in the temperature of hot body and the ambient is the temperature gradient for the heat loss by radiation. The radiation constant is calculated using the following equation:

$$Ms \frac{dq}{dt} = \alpha A \left(\left\{\frac{T_1}{100}\right\}^4 - \left\{\frac{T_2}{100}\right\}^4 \right) + \beta A (T_1 - T_2)^{1.23}$$

Where,

> M = Mass of the metal cylinder, w g; s = Specific heat of the metal, J/Kg.K; (dq/dt) = rate of heat loss by metal cylinder, W/s; T_1 = temperature of the metal body, K; T_2 = temperature of the ambient (Room Temperature), K; α = Radiation constant, W/m².K⁴ ; β = Convection factor; A = Surface area for heat transfer, m².

The parameters mentioned in the equation (02) are evaluated by different methods and substituted for calculating **α**.

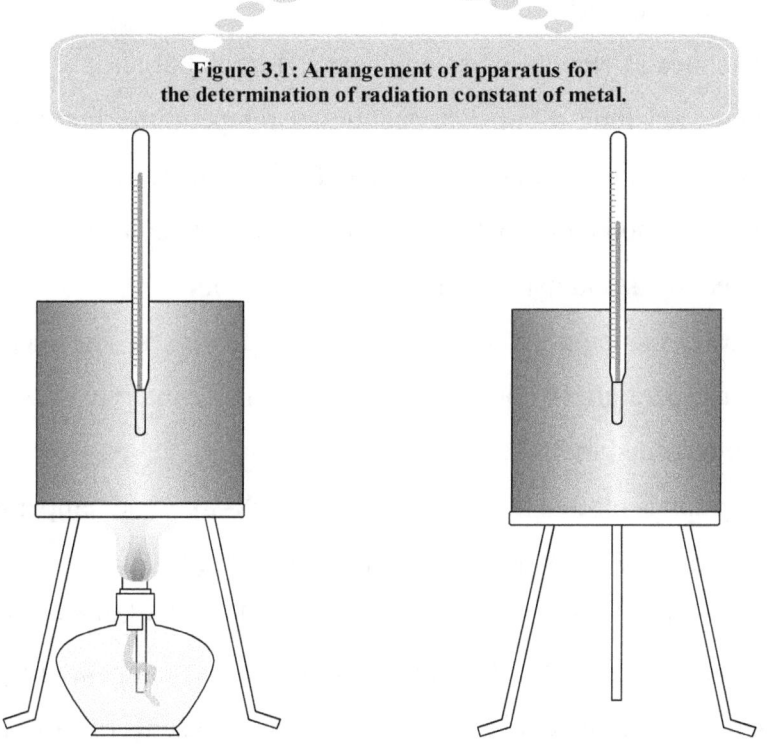

Figure 3.1: Arrangement of apparatus for the determination of radiation constant of metal.

Pharmaceutical Engineering Experimental Lab Manual-I (Unit Operations)

REQUIREMENTS

Metal cylinder (Iron), glass tripod stand, thermometer (360°C).

PROCEDURE

Arrangement of apparatus for the determination of radiation constant of a metal cylinder is shown in **Figure-3.1**.

1. A Metal (Iron) cylinder is cleaned and weighed (w g) thrice. The average weight is noted in **Table-3.1**.
2. The diameter and height of the cylinder are measured thrice. The average values are calculated. The radius of the cylinder is calculated. The surface area of the cylinder is calculated and recorded in **Table-3.1**.
3. The metal cylinder is heated using a Bunsen burner.
4. After reaching a constant maximum temperature, hot body is transferred to the glass tripod stand using long tongs.
5. The thermometer (360°C) is placed in a central hole cylinder and fixed to a stand using a thread (**Figure-3.1**).
6. Slowly the temperature of the hot body decreases. The decrease in temperature is noted in every five-minute interval. The data are recorded in **Table-3.2**.
7. A graph is plotted taking time (min.) on X-axis and temperature (°C) on Y-axis. Normally, a curve is observed.
8. Depending on the temperature at which the radiation constant is to be determined, a tangent is drawn at that temperature. The slope of the tangent is calculated, which represents rate of fall of

| Section-II | Expt-3: Radiation Constant of Iron Cylinder |

temperature. This parameter is related to rate of loss of heat (dq/dt) by the hot body (Iron).

9. Radiation constant (**α**) is determined at that temperature (Figure given in example).

PRECAUTIONS

- The metal cylinder should not be touched with hands.
- Care should be taken while transferring the hot Iron cylinder from the metal tripod to the glass tripod.

OBSERVATIONS AND CALCULATIONS:

At room temperature:

Wet bulb temperature = _____ °C _____ K

Dry bulb temperature = _____ °C _____ K

Table 3.1: Parameters of The Iron Cylinder

S. No	Parameters of the metal cylinder	Trial			Average in CGS system	Average in SI system
		1	2	3		
1	Weight, w g					
2	Diameter, d cm					
3	Radius, r cm					
4	Height, h cm					
5	Surface Area, A					

Specific heat (s):

Iron, s = 448 J/Kg.K; copper, s = 385 J/Kg.K; Brass, s = 370 J/Kg.K; Aluminium, s = 913 J/Kg.K

(Specific Heat Capacity is the heat needed to raise the temperature of 1 kg of the substance by 1K (or by 1°C))

Table 3.2: Radiation constant of a metal- Time Vs Temp.Plot

Time, min	Temp, °C	Time, min	Temp, °C	Time, min	Temp, °C	Time, min	Temp, °C

Report:

Radiation Constant of Iron, α =

Section-II Expt-3: Radiation Constant of Iron Cylinder

Example: 1

Calculate the radiation constant of iron at 80°C using the following:

M= 1840 g; s=448 J/Kg.K; D=6.2 cm;
T_1 = 80°C; T_2 = 28°C; h = 7.8 cm;
β = 2.8; α =?

Table 3.3: Radiation constant of a metal- Time Vs Temp.Plot

Time, t min	Temp, T °C	t min	T °C	t min	T °C	t min	T °C	t min	T °C	t min	T °C
0	306										
5	270	25	165	45	112	65	82	85	63	105	52
10	235	30	148	50	103	70	77	90	60	110	50
15	207	35	134	55	96	75	72	95	57	115	48
20	184	40	123	60	88	80	68	100	55	120	46

Solution:

The time-temperature profile is drawn on a graph paper using the given data (Figure).

A tangent (perpendicular line) is drawn using the following procedure:

At the point of desired temperature (80°C), two lines are drawn (A and B), on both sides of the point, intersecting the curve, using a protractor. From point A, curves are drawn on both sides of the curve. Using the same protractor, curves are drawn similarly from the point B, which intersect the above two curves at points C and D.

Points C and D are joined with a ruler. Using a setsquare, at 90°, a tangent (perpendicular line) is drawn on the curve. The slope of the tangent is calculated and found to be 1.1 (dq/dt).

Diameter of the iron cylinder, $D = 6.2$ cm or 0.062 m

Radius of the iron cylinder, $r = 6.2$ cm/2 $= 3.1$ cm or 0.031 m

Height (length) of the iron cylinder, $h = 7.8$ cm or 0.078 m

Surface area of the iron cylinder, $A = 2\pi r\ (r + h) = 2 \times 3.14 \times 0.031(0.031 + 0.078)$

$$= 0.1947 \times 0.109 = 0.0212\ m^2$$

Figure 3.2: Time – Temperature profile for calculating the slope of the tangent

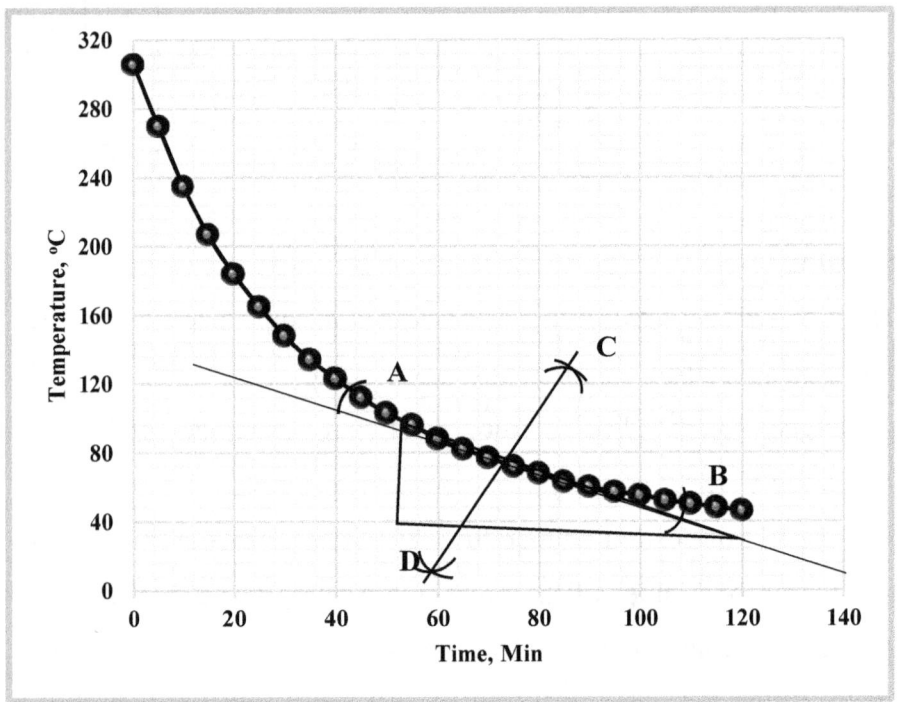

The other parameters are:

Section-II — Expt-3: Radiation Constant of Iron Cylinder

Mass of the iron cylinder, $M = 1840$ g or 1.84 kg;

Specific heat of iron cylinder, $s = 448$ J/Kg.K.

Room temperature, $T_2 = 28°C = 28 + 273.12 = 301.12$ K

Desired temperature, $T_1 = 80°C = 80 + 273.12 = 353.12$ K

Rate of Heat Transfer $(Q) = Q_c + Q_R$

Q_C = Rate of heat transfer/loss by conduction; Q_R = Rate of heat transfer/loss by Radiation;

$$Q = Ms \frac{dq}{dt}$$

Recall equation (2)

$$Ms \frac{dq}{dt} = \alpha A \left(\left\{\frac{T_1}{100}\right\}^4 - \left\{\frac{T_2}{100}\right\}^4\right) + \beta A (T_1-T_2)^{1.23}$$

$1.84 \times 448 \times 1.1 = \alpha \times 0.0212 \left(\left\{\frac{353.12}{100}\right\}^4 - \left\{\frac{301.12}{100}\right\}^4\right) + 2.8 \times 0.0212 (353.12-301.12)^{1.23}$

$906.752 = 0.0212 \, \alpha \, [(3.5312)^4 - (3.0112)^4] + 0.05936 (52)^{1.23}$

$906.752 = 0.0212 \, \alpha \, (155.4853 - 82.2164) + 0.05936 \times 129.0280$

$906.752 = \alpha \times 0.0212 \times 73.2689 + 7.6591$

$906.752 = 1.5533 \, \alpha + 7.6591$

$1.5533 \, \alpha = 906.752 - 7.6591 = 899.0929$

$\alpha = \dfrac{899.0929}{1.5533} = 578.8275$ J/min.m^2.K

or $\dfrac{578.8275}{60} = 9.647125$ J/s.m^2.K

$= 9.647125$ W/m². K

Example-02:

Diameter of the iron cylinder, $D = 1.5$ cm or 0.015 m

Radius of the iron cylinder, $r = 0.015$ cm/$2 = 0.0075$ m

Height (length) of the iron cylinder, $h = 0.06$ m

Surface area of the iron cylinder, $A = 2\pi r (r + h) = 2 \times 3.14 \times 0.0075$ $(0.0075 + 0.06)$

$$= 0.0471 \times 0.109 = 0.0675 \text{ m}^2$$

Mass of the iron cylinder, $M = 0.28$ kg;

Specific heat of iron cylinder, $s = 448$ J/Kg.K.

Room temperature, $T_2 = 28°C = 28 + 273.12 = 301.12$ K

Desired temperature, $T_1 = 80°C = 80 + 273.12 = 353.12$ K

The slope of the tangent is calculated and found to be 1 (dq/dt).

Time, t min	Temp, T °C	t min	T °C	t min	T °C	t min	T °C
0	240						
5	210	25	100	45	50	65	40
10	170	30	80	50	46	70	40
15	150	35	75	55	44	75	40
20	120	40	60	60	42		

$$Ms \frac{dq}{dt} = \alpha A \left(\left\{\frac{T_1}{100}\right\}^4 - \left\{\frac{T_2}{100}\right\}^4\right) + \beta A (T_1 - T_2)^{1.23}$$

$0.28 \times 448 \times 1.1 = \alpha \times 0.0675 \left(\left\{\frac{353.12}{100}\right\}^4 - \left\{\frac{301.12}{100}\right\}^4\right) + 2.8 \times 0.0675$ $(353.12 - 301.12)^{1.23}$

$125.44 = 0.0675 \alpha [(3.5312)^4 - (3.0112)^4] + 0.189 (52)^{1.23}$

125.44 = 0.0675 α (155.4853 - 82.2164) + 0.189 × 129.0280

125.44 = α 0.0675 × 73.2689 + 24.3862

125.44 = α 4.9456 + 24.3862

α 4.9456 = 125.44 - 24.3862

α 4.9456 = 101.0538

$$\alpha = \frac{101.0538}{4.9456} = 20.4330 \text{ J/min.m}^2\text{. K}$$

$$or \quad \frac{20.4330}{60} = 0.34055 \text{ J/s.m}^2\text{. K}$$

= 9.647125 W/m². K

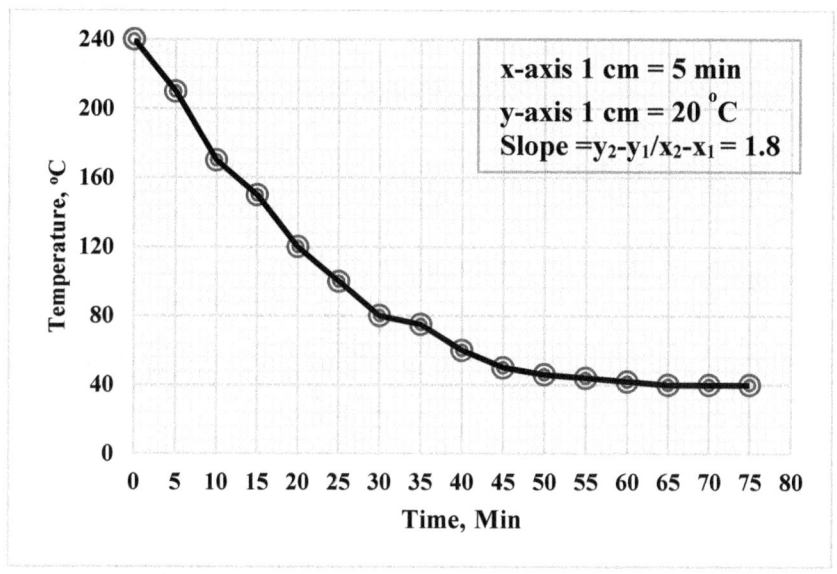

Figure 3.3: Time – Temperature profile for calculating the slope of the tangent

QUESTION BANK

1. State and explain Stefan-Boltzmann's law of heat transmission for radiation.
2. Define the term 'radiation'. Give one example.
3. Explain different modes of heat transfer with one example each.
4. Explain the principle involved in the determination of radiation constant of a metal.

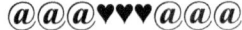

Expt-4: Determination of Radiation Constant of Brass Cylinder

AIM:

To determine the radiation constant of Brass cylinder

REQUIREMENTS:

Brass cylinder, thermometer, wooden plank, stop clock, Tongs & Heating source

PRINCIPLE:

Heat is lost from hot cylinder surface to surrounding atmosphere by means of conduction and radiation. Heat transfer by radiation occurs, energy transfer through space by means of electromagnetic radiation (waves). Thus, a body acts as an emitter, then energy being transmitted through the intervening spaces, and it is effective even in a perfect vacuum or inter-spacious space. The amount of thermal energy radiated by a surface is increased rapidly with increasing temperature, when a heat flows by actual mixing of warmer portions with cooler portions of the same material. This mechanism is known as **Convection**.

Stefan-Boltzmann law gives the total amount of radiation emitted by a body:

$$q = bAT^4$$

Where, q = energy radiated per second, W or J/s; A = Area of radiating surface, m²; T = Absolute temperature of the radiating surface, K; b = Constant, W/m². K⁴

The above equation, the rate of heating depends upon the temperature and surface area of the emitter and the absorption capacity of the material to be heated.

The difference in the temperature of hot body and the ambient is the temperature gradient for the heat loss by radiation. The radiation constant is calculated using the following equation:

$$Ms \frac{dq}{dt} = \alpha A \left(\left\{ \frac{T_1}{100} \right\}^4 - \left\{ \frac{T_2}{100} \right\}^4 \right) + \beta A (T_1 - T_2)^{1.23}$$

Where,

M = Mass of the metal cylinder, w g; s = Specific heat of the metal, J/Kg.K; (dq/dt) = rate of heat loss by metal cylinder, W/s; T_1 = temperature of the metal body, K; T_2 = temperature of the ambient (Room Temperature), K; α = Radiation constant, W/m².K⁴ ; β = Convection factor; A = Surface area for heat transfer, m².

Section-II   Expt-4: Radiation Constant of Brass Cylinder

REQUIREMENTS

Metal cylinder (Iron), glass tripod stand, thermometer (360°C).

PROCEDURE

A Metal (Brass) cylinder is cleaned and weighed (w, g) thrice. The average weight is noted in **Table-4.1**.

1. The diameter and height of the cylinder are measured thrice. The average values are calculated. The radius of the cylinder is calculated. The surface area of the cylinder is calculated and recorded in **Table-4.1**.
2. The metal cylinder is heated using a Bunsen burner.
3. After reaching a constant maximum temperature, hot body is transferred to the glass tripod stand using long tongs.
4. The thermometer (360°C) is placed in a central hole cylinder and fixed to a stand using a thread.
5. Slowly the temperature of the hot body decreases. The decrease in temperature is noted in every five-minute interval. The data are recorded in **Table-4.2**.
6. A graph is plotted taking time (min.) on X- axis and temperature (°C) on Y-axis. Normally, a curve is observed.
7. Depending on the temperature at which the radiation constant is to be determined, a tangent is drawn at that temperature. The slope of the tangent is calculated, which represents rate of fall of temperature. This parameter is related to rate of loss of heat (dq/dt) by the hot body (Brass).

8. Radiation constant (α) of Brass is determined at that temperature.

OBSERVATIONS AND CALCULATIONS:

At room temperature:

Wet bulb temperature = _____ °C _____ K

Dry bulb temperature = _____ °C _____ K

Table 4.1: Parameters of the Brass cylinder

S.No	Parameters of the Brass cylinder	Trial			Average in CGS system	Average in SI system
		1	2	3		
1	Weight, w g					
2	Diameter, d cm					
3	Radius, r cm					
4	Height, h cm					
5	Surface Area, A					

Specific heat (s): Brass, s = 370 J/Kg.K;

Table 4.2: Radiation constant of a brass-Time Vs Temp. Plot Data

Time, min	Temp, °C	Time, min	Temp, °C	Time, min	Temp, °C	Time, min	Temp, °C

REPORT:

The Radiation Constant of Brass cylinder, α was found to be = _____ W/m². K.

Expt-5: Determination of Radiation Constant of Unpainted and Painted Glass

AIM

To determine the radiation constant of glass (unpainted and painted).

THEORY

Heat transfer by radiation involves the transfer of energy in the form of electromagnetic waves. Along with radiation, convection and conduction mechanisms also operate in heat transfer. These become significant at higher temperatures.

All solid bodies radiate energy when their temperatures are above absolute zero. The principle form of radiant energy on industrial applications is thermal energy. Therefore, this is known as thermal energy.

The radiant energy emitted by a hot body is expressed by Stefan-Boltzmann law as given below:

$$q = bAT^4$$

Section-II Expt-5: Radiation Constant of Unpainted and Painted Glass

Where, q = energy radiated per second, W (or J/s) A = area of radiating surface, m^2; T = absolute temperature of the radiating surface, K b = constant, W/m^{2}xK^4

Stefan-Boltzmann law is applicable to a 'black body'. However, it can also be applied to 'grey body', in order to obtain a rough estimate of the constant. According to above equation, the rate of heating depends upon the temperature and surface area of the emitting body. At the same time, it also depends upon the absorption capacity of the material to be heated. This characteristic is evaluated.

The difference in the temperature of hot body and the ambient is the temperature gradient for the heat loss by radiation. The radiation constant is calculated using the following equation:

Total heat lost by the body	=	Heat loss due to radiation	+	Heat loss due to convection

$$(M_1 s_1 - M_2 s_2) \frac{dq}{dt} = \alpha A \left(\left\{ \frac{T_1}{100} \right\}^4 - \left\{ \frac{T_2}{100} \right\}^4 \right) + \beta A (T_1 - T_2) \ldots (03)$$

Where,

M_1 = mass of water, w kg; M_2 = mass of round bottom flask (unpainted/painted), kg; s_1 = specific heat of water, J/kg.K; s_2 = specific heat of glass, J/kg.K; (dq/dt) = rate of heat loss by the apparatus, W/s; T_1 = temperature of the metal body, K; T_2 = temperature of the ambient (room), K; α = radiation constant, $W/m^2.K^4$; β = convection factor; A = surface area for heat transfer, m^2

Figure 5.1. Arrangement of apparatus for the determination of radiation constant of glass (unpainted)

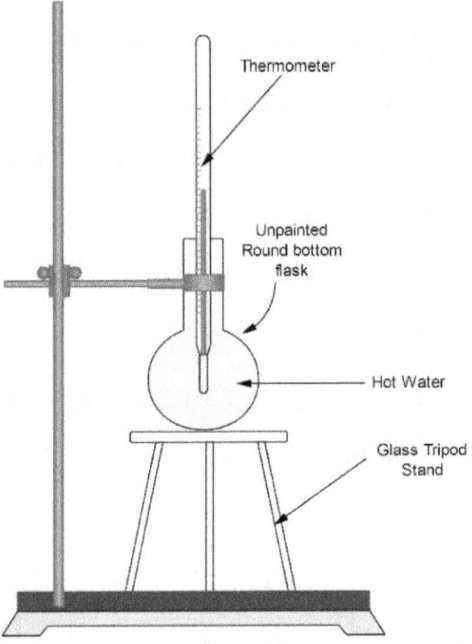

The parameters mentioned in equation (3) are evaluated by different methods and substituted for calculating a. The arrangement of apparatus is shown in **Figure 5.1**.

The special feature of the heat transmission by radiation is that radiant energy penetrates to a certain distance in the material. Beyond a particular point, heat transfer by radiation becomes ineffective. For this reason, formation of surface skin must be avoided. When glass apparatus is painted with silver oxide (white or

Section-II   Expt-5: Radiation Constant of Unpainted and Painted Glass

any other colour), the rate of radiation decreases, because painting act as insulation by radiation.

REQUIREMENTS

Round bottom flask with long neck, 500 ml; Hotplate or burner; Thermometer, 110°C; Glass tripod stand; Painted (white colored) round bottom flask with long neck; Painted (green coloured) round bottom flask with long neck.

PROCEDURE

Arrangement of apparatus for the determination of radiation constant of unpainted glass apparatus is shown in **Figure-5.1**.

1. A round bottom flask (unpainted) is cleaned and dried.
2. The weight of the flask is determined *(M_2 kg)* and reported in **Table 5.1**.
3. The diameter *(D)* of the round bottom flask is determined and reported in **Table 5.1**.
4. The diameter *(d)* of neck of the flask is determined and reported in **Table 5.1**.
5. Boiled hot water is prepared and a measured volume of hot water is transferred to the flask carefully. The volume of water is recorded (M_1). The external surface of the round bottom flask is thoroughly dried and cleaned. The flask with hot water is placed on the tripod stand (**Figure 5.1**).

6. Thermometer (110 °C) is dipped to the center of the flask and tied at the top to an iron stand.
7. Slowly the temperature of the hot body decreases. The decrease in temperature is noted every minute. The data are recorded in **Table 5.1**.
8. A graph is plotted by taking time (minute) on x-axis and temperature on y-axis. Normally a curve is obtained.
9. Depending on the temperature at which radiation constant is determined, a tangent is drawn at that temperature. The slope is calculated. This parameter is related to the rate of heat loss *(dq/dt)*.
10. Radiation constant (a) is determined at that temperature.
11. The same procedure is repeated with round bottom flask painted with silver oxide (white colour) and green colour.

Precautions:

(1) The glass surface should not be touched with hands while taking readings.

(2) Care should be taken while transferring hot water quantitatively into the round bottom flask.

Observations and Calculations

At room temperature: Wet bulb temperature = _____ °C

Dry bulb temperature = _____ °C

Section-II   Expt-5: Radiation Constant of Unpainted and Painted Glass

Table 5.1: Parameters of the Glass Apparatus for Heat Transfer

Sl. No.	Parameter of the metal cylinder	Trial 1	Trial 2	Trial 3	Average in CGS system	Average in SI system
1	Weight, M_1 g					
2	Diameter, d					
3	Radius, r cm	—	—	—		
4	Height, h cm					
5	Surface area,	—	—	—		

Volume of hot water transferred, M_2 = ____ ml or _____ g or kg
Heat loss by convection, $\beta = 0$; Specific heat of water, $s_1 = 4190$ J/kg.K; Specific heat of glass (flint), $s_2 = 500$ J/kg.K

Table 5.2: Radiation Constant of a Metal-Time Vs. Temp. Plot Data

Time, min	Temp, °C	Time, min	Temp, °C	Time, min	Temp, °C	Time, min	Temp, °C

REPORT:

Radiation constant of glass, α =

(unpainted/white painted/green painted)

Example:

Calculate the radiation constant (a) of the glass at 75°C using the following data:

M_1 = 565 ml; M_2 = 129.5 g; T_2 = 27°C; T_1 = 75°C; dq/dt = 0.66; β = 2.8; s_1 = 4190 J/Kg.K,

s_2 = 500 J/Kg.K; Diameter of round bottom flask = 10.6 cm; Diameter of neck of flask = 3.1 cm

Solution:

Diameter of the round bottom flask, D = 10.6 cm or 0.106 m

Radius of the round bottom flask, R = 10.6 cm/2 = 5.3 cm or 0.053 m Diameter of neck of the flask, d = 3.1 cm or 0.031 m; Radius of neck of the flask, r = 3.1/2 cm or 1.55 cm or 0.0155 m Surface area of the round bottom flask = $4\pi R^2 - \pi r^2$

$$= 4 \times 3.14 \times (0.053)^2 - 3.14 (0.0155)^2$$

$$= 0.03531 - 0.00077$$

$$= 0.03454 \text{ m}^2.$$

Section-II Expt-5: Radiation Constant of Unpainted and Painted Glass

The other parameters are:

M_1 = 565 ml/min or 0.565 g or 0.565 kg; M_2 = 129.5 g/min or 0.1295 kg; Room temperature, T_2 = 27°C = 27 + 273.12 = 300.12 K; Desired temperature, T_1 = 75°C = 75 + 273.12 = 348.12 K

Recall equation (3)

$$(M_1 s_1 - M_2 s_2) \frac{dq}{dt} = \alpha A \left(\left\{ \frac{T_1}{100} \right\}^4 - \left\{ \frac{T_2}{100} \right\}^4 \right) + \beta A (T_1 - T_2) \ldots$$

(03)

$(0.565 \times 4190 + 0.1295 \times 500)0.66 =$

$\alpha \times 0.03454 \left(\left\{ \frac{348.12}{100} \right\}^4 - \left\{ \frac{300.12}{100} \right\}^4 \right) + 2.8 \times 0.03454(348.12 - 300.12)$

$(224.65 + 64.75)0.66 = 0.03454 \, \alpha \, [(3.4812)^4 - (3.0012)^4]) + 0.09672(48)^{1.23}$

$2306.4 \times 0.66 = 0.03454 \, \alpha \, (146.86 - 81.13) + 0.09675 \times 116.93$

$1522.224 = \alpha \times 0.03454 \times 65.73 + 11.3095$

$1522.224 = 22.703 \, \alpha + 11.3095$

$22.703 \, \alpha = 1522.22 - 11.3095 = 1510.91$

$a = \dfrac{1510.91}{22.703} = 66.55$ J/min.m². K $or \ \dfrac{66.50}{60} = 1.108$ J/s.m². K

$= 1.108$ W/m². K

QUESTION BANK

1. Describe the principle involved in the determination of radiation constant of glass.
2. What is the effect of painting on glass on the radiation constant?

@@@♥♥@@@

Expt-6: Determination of Overall Heat Transfer Coefficients.

AIM:

To determine the overall heat transfer coefficient of a heat exchanger (glass cylinder/insulated glass cylinder).

THEORY

Heat transfer by convection is involved between two liquids, when these are separated by glass wall. The differences in the modes of feeding largely determine the efficiency of a heat process. When the hot fluid and the cold fluid enter the apparatus from the same end, the flow is parallel to each other. This arrangement is known as *parallel flow*. When the feed of hot fluid is passed through one end of the apparatus, while the cold fluid is passed through the other end, this arrangement is known as *counter-current* or *counter flow* method.

The above types of flow are observed in a heat exchanger.

Heat exchangers are the devices used for transferring heat from one fluid (hot gas or steam) to another fluid (liquid) through a metal wall.

Some heat exchanger (or heater) equipment are:

-Tubular heater (shell-and-tube heater)

-Multipass heater

-Two-pass floating head heater

In a heat exchanger, the overall heat transfer coefficient will be nearer to the cold liquid side (because it is smaller of the two coefficients). The efficiency of a heat exchanger can be improved by passing the liquid at a high velocity.

APPLICATIONS:

Most of the chemical and pharmaceutical industries employ a variety of heat transfer equipment. Some of the processes, which involve heat transfer in pharmacy are:

- Preparation of starch paste for granulation
- Crystallization
- Evaporation
- Distillation

In industrial process, heat energy is transferred by various methods.

PRINCIPLE

When the feed of hot fluid is passed through one end of the apparatus and the cold fluid is passed through the other end, this arrangement is known as *counter-current* or *counter flow* method.

The overall heat transfer coefficient of a glass tube is mathematically expressed for a counter current flow as:

$$U = Q/A \times \Delta t_{av} \qquad (4)$$

Where, Q = amount of heat transferred, W (J/s); A = surface area of the glass tube, m^2; Δt = temperature gradient, K; U = overall heat transfer coefficient, W/m^2. K;

In equation (4), the term Q is represented as:

$$Q = Q_1 + Q_2 / 2 \qquad (5)$$

where Q_1 = heat loss by steam, W (J.s); Q_2 = heat gain by cold body, W (J.s)

Heat loss by hot body may be expressed as:

$$Q_1 = M_1.L + M_1.s.t_1 \qquad (6)$$

and heat gain by the cold body may be expressed as:

$Q_2 = M_2.s.t_2$

Where, M_1 = mass of condensed steam, kg, M_2 = mass of circulating water, kg; s = specific heat of steam. J/kg.K; L = latent heat of vaporization of water, J/kg; t_1 = temperature drop on steam, K;= temperature rise on the circulating water side, K

The temperature gradient. Δt_{av} is expressed as: $\Delta t_{av} = \Delta t_1 + \Delta t_2 / 2$

Where, Δt_1 = difference in temperature on steam side, K; Δt_2 = difference in temperatures on cold water side, K

The water condenser used in the laboratory for distillation is an example for the counter current flow of liquids and heat transfer. Thus, overall all heat transfer coefficient is determined using water condenser. Water condenser (without wounding with cotton rope, insulating) and non-insulated glass condenser can be used. These differences reflect the heat transfer efficiency of a condenser.

The cold water is circulated through the jacket of the water condenser (**Figure-6.1**). As a result, the steam in the condenser gets condensed, due to heat transfer by conduction through the glass wall, followed by convection. Thus, the condensed water is collected at the other end.

Figure 6.1: Arrangement of apparatus and counter current flow of liquids is shown

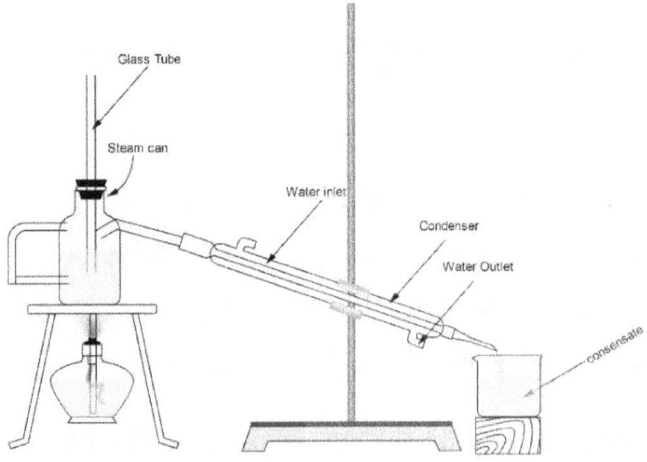

Section-II Expt-6: Overall Heat Transfer Coefficients

REQUIREMENTS

Steam generator; Water condenser (non-insulated); Thermometer, 110°C; Water condenser (insulated); Bent tube.

PROCEDURE

The assembly of apparatus is shown in the **Figure-6.1**.

1. The length and diameter of the plain water condenser is determined and reported in the observations. Based on these values, surface area of the condenser is estimated.
2. Using the plain water condenser, the distillation apparatus is assembled as shown in **Figure-6.1**.
3. The inlet of water condenser is connected to the tap. The outlet of the condenser is placed in the beaker (2-liter beaker).
4. The temperature of the water at the inlet of the condenser is noted. This will be same as the temperature of the tap water. The temperature is reported in **Table 6.1**.
5. The steam generator is heated so that steam will be generated. After some time, the thermometer shows constant temperature. The temperature is noted **(Table 6.1)** and experiment is started from the point. The steam passes through the water condenser and gets condensed in the condenser due to circulation of water in the jacket.
6. The condensate gets collected into the beaker (50 ml).
7. Allow the experiment for 2 minutes (after attaining constant temperature of steam).

8. The quantity of condensate water is collected and its temperature is noted.

9. The quantity of circulated water is collected at the outlet of condenser and its temperature is noted (Table 6.1).

The entire experiment is repeated by replacing the plain water con-denser with an insulated water condenser.

Precautions: (1) The rate of flow of water through the jacket of the water condenser must be maintained constant. (2) The joints in the assembly of apparatus must be as short as possible, so as to prevent the heat loss at these points.

OBSERVATIONS AND CALCULATIONS

Observations with Plain Water Condenser

Diameter of the condenser, d = _____ cm = _____

Radius of the condenser, r = _____ cm = _____

Length of the condenser, l = _____ cm = _____

Area of the condenser, $A = 2\pi r l$

Latent heat of vaporization of water, $L = 226.1$ J/kg

Specific heat of steam, $s = 4190$ J/kg. K

The following calculations are made. Recall equations (5) and (6)

Heat loss by steam, $Q_1 = M_1 . L + M_1 . s . \Delta t_1$

Heat gain by tap water, $Q_2 = M_2 . s . t_2$

Heat transferred, $Q = Q_1 + Q_2 / 2$

Recall equation (4),

Section-II — Expt-6: Overall Heat Transfer Coefficients

$U = Q/A \times \Delta t_{av}$

Similar observations can be obtained by conducting the experiment using insulated water jacket condenser.

REPORT

Overall heat transfer coefficient of plain glass tube (water condenser) =

Overall heat transfer coefficient of insulated glass tube =

Inference:

The heat transfer coefficient of the insulated glass tube is higher/lower than the plain glass tube.

TABLE 6.1: Parameters for Counter Current Flow

	Water condenser Circulating water		On steam side of the condenser	
	Tap water	Water outlet	Steam	Condensate
Temperature, °C				
Temperature, K				
Difference in temperatures	Δt_1		Δt_2	
Average temperature, Δt_{av}	$\dfrac{\Delta t_1 + \Delta t_2}{2}$			
Volume of water in 2 minutes	-	M_2	-	M_1
Mass of water in 2 minutes, kg				
Mass of water per second, kg/s				

Pharmaceutical Engineering Experimental Lab Manual-I (Unit Operations)

Example:
Calculate the overall heat transfer coefficient of glass water condenser (heat exchanger) using the following data.

$D = 4$ cm; $l = 34.1$ cm;
Steam temperature = 95°C; Condensate temperature 44°C
Temperature of cold water (tap water) = 27°C;
Circulating water, outlet temperature = 48°C
Volume of water circulating, M_2 = 930 ml/2 minutes
Volume of condensate, M_1 = 17 ml/2 minutes
Specific heat of water, s = 4190 J/kg.K
Latent heat of vaporization, L = 226.1 J/kg

Solution:
Data:
d = 4 cm or 0.04 m; r = 0.02 m L = 34.1 cm or 0.341 m; Area = $2\pi r$
= 2 x 3.14 x 0.02 x 0.314 = 0.0429 m²
M_1 = 17 ml/2 min or 0.017 kg/2 min or 0.017/60 x 2 kg/s = 0.0001417 kg/s
M_2 = 930 ml/2 min. or 930 g/2 min or 0.930 kg/2 min = 0.930/2 x 60 kg/s = 0.00775 kg/s

Steam side:
Steam temperature = 95°C = 95 +273.12 = 368.12 K
Condensate temperature = 44°C = 44 + 273.12 = 317.12 K
Difference in temperatures on steam side, Δt_1 = 368.12 - 317.12 = 51 K

Cold water side:
Tap water temperature = 27°C = 27 + 273.12 = 300.12 K
Circulating water temperature = 48°C = 48 + 273.12 = 321.12 K
Difference in temperatures on cold water side, Δt_2 = 321.12 - 300.12 = 21 K
Average temperature, = Δt_{av} = Δt_1 + Δt_2 / 2 = 51 + 21 / 2 = 72/ 2 = 36 K

$M_1 = 0.0001417$ kg/s; $M_2 = 0.00775$ kg/s

Heat loss by steam, $Q_1 = M_1 \cdot L + M_1 \cdot s \cdot t_1$
  $= 0.0001417 \times 226.1 + 0.0001417 \times 4190 \times 51$
  $= 0.0320 + 30.280 = 30.312$ J/s

Heat gain by tap water, $Q_2 = M_2 \cdot s \cdot t_2 = 0.0077 \times 4190 \times 21 = 677.523$ J/s

Heat transferred, $Q = Q_1 + Q_2 / 2 = 30.312 + 677.523/ 2 = 707.835/2$
$= 353.92$ J/s

  Recall equation (4)
  $U = Q/A \times \Delta t_{av} = 353.92/ 0.0429 \times 36 = 353.92 / 1.5444 = 229.16$ J/s.kg.K $= 229.16$ W/kg.K

QUESTION BANK

1. What is meant by overall heat transfer coefficient? What is its significance?
2. Compare the heat transmission following counter current and parallel current feed techniques with relevant equations.

SECTION-III
EVAPORATION

Expt-7: Determination of Factors Affecting Rate of Evaporation

AIM:

To study the effect of various factors affecting rate of evaporation

THEORY

Evaporation is a process of vaporizing large quantities of volatile liquid to get a concentrated product. Evaporation is a surface phenomenon, i.e., mass transfer takes place from the surface. Thus, no boiling occurs. The practical definition of evaporation is the removal of solvent from the solution by heating the liquor in a suitable vessel and withdrawing the vapour, leaving a concentrated liquid residue in the vessel.

Different forms of liquids like solutions or suspensions can be subjected to evaporation. The condition is that the liquid must be volatile, while the solute must be nonvolatile. Although the focus in most of the evaporation processes is in collecting concentrated product, sometimes evaporating solvent needs to be recovered for the reasons of its toxicity, cost etc.

Applications:

Evaporation process is used in pharmaceutical practice, pharmaceutical industries, chemical industries etc. for the manufacture of bulk drugs. This process is used in the preparation of insulin, penicillin G, blood plasma etc.

PRINCIPLE

The rate of evaporation depends on several factors such as temperature, viscosity, concentration of the slurry, vapour pressure, surface area, time of evaporation, films, and deposits. Moisture content of the feed, type of product required, and economic factors also influence the evaporation.

a. The higher the temperature, the greater will be the rate of evaporation. Rate of evaporation is directly proportional to the vapour pressure of the liquid.

b. The greater the surface area of the liquid, the greater will be the evaporation. For this reason, evaporation is conducted in evaporators with large heating surface area. This is verified by taking beakers of different surface area, i.e., 50 ml, 100 ml capacity. When same quantity of slurry (or water) is maintained and exposed to same time and same temperature, the differences in the initial and final weights permit the verification of factor, surface area. Rate of evaporation can be used as a tool for the verification of surface area factor.

c. If the time of exposure is longer, greater will be the evaporation.

d. Films and deposits formed during evaporation reduce the evaporation.

e. Higher the viscosity of the slurry, the lower the rate of evaporation. This is verified by taking slurries of different viscosities and subjecting to evaporation at constant temperature and constant surface area. For this purpose, glycerin-water mixtures of different glycerin concentration, by maintaining same volume of slurry. In other words, the slurries have different viscosities. Rate of evaporation can be used as a tool for the verification of the effect of viscosity.

f. Higher the concentration of dissolved solids, the lower the rate of evaporation. This is verified by taking slurries of different concentrations of dissolved solids (for example, sodium chloride) at constant temperature, constant surface area, and constant volume of slurry. The working concentrations of sodium chloride do not significantly alter the viscosity factor. Rate of evaporation can be used as a tool for the verification of concentration factor.

REQUIREMENTS

Beaker, 50 ml; Glycerin; Beaker, 100 ml; Purified water; Beaker, 250 ml; Sodium chloride

Water-bath; Balance; Weight box; Measuring scale; Measuring cylinder;

Section-III   Expt-7: Factors Affecting Rate of Evaporation

PROCEDURE

The effect of surface area, viscosity, and concentration of the solution are studied.

Effect of surface area:

1. Beakers measuring 50 ml, 100 ml, and 250 ml are cleaned.
2. 25 ml quantity of water is taken in each beaker.
3. Beakers containing water are weighed. The weights are recorded in column 3 of **Table-7.1**. (Initial weight of beaker, w_1 g).
4. All the beakers containing water are heated in a water bath at constant temperature (70°C) for 30 minutes.
5. After heating, all the beakers are weighed again. The weights are recorded in column 4 of **Table-7.1**. (Final weight of beaker, w_2 g).
6. The difference between the weights is determined, w g. The difference reflects the amount of water evaporated during 30 minutes.
7. Radius of the beaker is noted. Using the radius, surface area of beakers is calculated using the below mentioned formula and is recorded in column 2 of **Table-7.1**.
   Surface area of beaker = πr^2
8. Rate of evaporation is calculated using the following formula:

   Rate of evaporation = Quantity of water evaporated (w) / Time of heating in minutes = _____ **g/min**

9. A graph is plotted by taking rate of evaporation on *y-axis* and surface area on *x-axis*.

Effect of viscosity:

1. Different concentrations of glycerin and water mixtures are prepared in different beakers as shown in the following table:

Glycerin	Water	Concentration
5 ml	45 ml	10%
10 ml	40 ml	20%
15 ml	35 ml	30%
20 ml	30 ml	40%

2. The beakers containing glycerin—water mixtures are weighed (w_3 g). Viscosities of these mixtures at room temperature are given in column 3 of **Table-7.2**. Weights are recorded in column 5 of **Table-7.2**.
3. All the beakers are heated in a water–bath at constant temperature (70°C) for 30 minutes.
4. All the beakers are weighed again after heating (w_4 g). Weights are recorded in column 6 of **Table-7.2**.
5. The difference between the weights is determined. The difference reflects the amount of water evaporated during 30 minutes.
6. Rate of evaporation is calculated.
7. A graph is plotted by taking rate of evaporation on *y-axis* and viscosity on *x-axis*.

Effect of concentration:

1. 2, 4, 6, and 8% w/v solutions of sodium chloride are prepared by dissolving 1, 2, 3, and 4 g of sodium chloride in 50 ml of water in beakers.
2. The beakers containing sodium chloride solutions are weighed (w_5 g). Weights are recorded in column 4 of **Table-7.3**.
3. All the beakers are heated in water — bath at constant temperature (70°C) for 30 minutes.
4. All the beakers are weighed again after heating (w_6 g). Weights are recorded in column 5 of **Table-7.3**.
5. The difference between the weights is determined. The difference reflects the amount of water evaporated during 30 minutes.
6. Rate of evaporation is calculated.
7. A graph is plotted by taking rate of evaporation on *y-axis* and concentration on *x-axis*.

OBSERVATIONS AND CALCULATIONS

TABLE 7.1: Effect of Surface Area

Sl. No.	Surface area of beaker, cm²	Initial weight of beaker, W_1 g	Final weight of beaker, W_2 g	Difference in weights, w g
				(3) - (4)
(1)	(2)	(3)	(4)	(5)
1.				
2.				
3.				

Time of heating, min	Rate of evaporation, g/min
	(5)/ (6)
(6)	(7)

TABLE 7.2: Effect of Viscosity

Sl. No.	Concern-ration of glycerin-water mixture	Viscosity of glycerin-water mixture	Initial weight of beaker, w_3 g	Final weight of beaker, w_4 g
(1)	(2)	(3)	(4)	(5)
1	10%	1.2823		
2	20%	1.8765		
3	30%	2.4020		
4	40%	2.9829		

Difference in weights, Weights, w g	Time of heating, g/min	Rate of evaporation
(3) - (4)		(6)/ (7)
(6)	(7)	(8)

TABLE 7.3: Effect of Concentration

Sl. No.	Content-ration of sodium chloride solution	Initial weight of beaker + solution, w_s g	Final weight of beaker + solution, w, g
(1)	(2)	(3)	(4)
1	2%		
2	4%		
3	6%		
4	8%		

Difference in weights, w g	Time of heating, min	Rate of evaporation, g/min
(3)-(4)		(5)/(6)
(5)	(6)	(7)

REPORT:

With increase in surface area, rate of evaporation_____.

With increase in viscosity of the solution, rate of evaporation_____.

With increase in concentration of sodium chloride solution, rate of evaporation_____.

QUESTION BANK

1. Define evaporation.
2. Describe the factors affecting evaporation.
3. Illustrate a few examples where evaporation phenomenon is used in pharmaceutical industry.
4. Enumerate applications of evaporation.
5. What is the principle involved in evaluating the factors affecting rate of evaporation?

@@@♥♥@@@

SECTION-IV
DISTILLATION

Expt-8: Preparation of Azeotropic Alcohol-Azeotropic Distillation

AIM:

To prepare absolute alcohol from rectified spirit by azeotropic distillation using glycerin.

THEORY

Azeotropic mixture is the solution that distils unchanged at a constant temperature. Such solutions are also known as *constant boiling mixtures.* An example of this type is 89.43 mol % mixture of ethanol and water at atmospheric pressure. In a mixture, if the volatilities of the components are equal, the mixture has a relative volatility of 1.0. Hence, further purification cannot be obtained by conventional distillation. These solutions deviate the Raoult's law to a large extent. Hence, azeotropic distillation is employed.

Azeotropic mixtures are of two types:

Minimum boiling point azeotropic solution:

This is a type of azeotropic mixture with a maximum vapour pressure or minimum boiling point. These systems are known as Type II solutions. Examples are: (i) chloroform and acetone; (ii) water and nitric acid.

Maximum boiling point azeotropic solution:

This is a type of azeotropic mixture with a minimum vapour pressure or maximum boiling point. These systems are known as Type III solutions.

Examples are: (i) water and ethanol; (ii) benzene and ethanol)

Applications:

The liquor from fermentation process is a common source of ethanol in a concentration of approximately 8 to 10%. Absolute alcohol can be obtained by azeotropic distillation.

The advantage of this method is that a simple distillation apparatus can be used.

PRINCIPLE

Azeotropic solutions (or constant boiling solutions) cannot be completely separated by simple, steam, vacuum, or fractional distillations, because both the vapour and the liquid (in the still) have a mixture of components. Such a mixture can be separated by azeotropic distillation.

Azeotropic distillation is a distillation method in which azeotropic mixture is broken by the addition of a third substance that forms a new azeotrope with one of the components.

The relative volatility of the individual components can be changed by adding a third substance. For example, glycerin is added to the azeotropic mixture of water and ethyl alcohol (rectified spirit). Glycerin breaks the water-alcohol mixture forming a new azeotrope, glycerin and water (because both are more polar than alcohol). Therefore, the volatility of ethyl alcohol (comparatively less polar liquid) enhances. On distillation, ethyl alcohol distils freely leaving behind water and glycerin in the still. This process continues' until all alcohol is completely distilled (at a temperature of 78.3°C). Therefore, practically absolute ethyl alcohol can be obtained from the azeotropic distillation.

When benzene is added to ethyl alcohol-water mixture, the reverse phenomenon is observed. The new azeotrope is benzene-alcohol (relatively less polar) and water becomes free that can be distilled off in pure form. Then the azeotrope breaks further giving benzene as condensate. Thus, absolute alcohol remains in the still.

REQUIREMENTS

Distillation flask, 250 ml; Glycerin with side tube; Distilled water; Two holed rubber cork; Rectified spirit; Thermometer, 110°C; Safety tube; Water condenser; Receiving adaptor; Beaker, 100 ml; Specific gravity bottle, 10 ml; Balance; Measuring cylinder, 100 ml; Bunsen burner; Stands.

PROCEDURE

Assembling of apparatus:

The apparatus is assembled as shown the **Figure 8.1**. To facilitate assembling, detailed description is given here.

1. 250 ml round bottom flask is fitted to two holed rubber cork.
2. Through one hole of rubber cork, thermometer is placed. Thermometer is positioned such that the tip of the thermometer should be exactly in front of the side tube. With this arrangement, thermometer shows exact temperature of vapours (boiling point).
3. Through the other hole, safety tube is placed. It facilitates free escape of excess pressure inside, if builds up.
4. To the side tube, water condenser is attached with the help of rubber cork. Water condenser is inclined towards receiver. This position is helpful for free forward movement of condensed liquid.
5. The other end of condenser is connected to the receiving adaptor.

6. The inlet of the water condenser is connected to water tap and outlet is left open into the sink. Water is introduced counter current to the flow of vapour.
7. A receiver (beaker) is placed below the adaptor. (Alternatively receiving adaptor with side tube can be connected to ground glass flask tightly).

METHOD:

Careful attention is required while handling all glass --distillation apparatus.

1. Fifty ml of rectified spirit (alcohol) and 30 ml of water are mixed. This mixture is placed in the distillation flask.
2. Fifteen ml of glycerin is added to the above mixture. The three-component mixture is formed in the round bottom flask.
3. The flask is heated continuously with the help of a Bunsen burner. The mixture gets heated and after some time starts boiling.
4. The temperature is noted at which alcohol distils. This temperature remains constant and is recorded.
5. Alcohol vapour condenses in the condenser and gets collected in the receiver. Collection of condensate is stopped when temperature (in thermometer) rises suddenly. This point indicates that distillation of alcohol is completed and the beginning of distillation of a new azeotrope (Glycerin - Water).

Section-IV Expt-8: Azeotropic Distillation

6. The volume of absolute alcohol collected is measured and recorded.
7. Specific gravity of alcohol (collected) is calculated using the model calculation shown. While taking the weights, alcohol and water should be maintained a temperature of 25°C by keeping the containers of these solvents in water bath. If temperature is not maintained, erroneous results are possible.
8. Per cent purity of alcohol is determined by comparing the specific gravity of alcohol with that of the standard values given in IP.

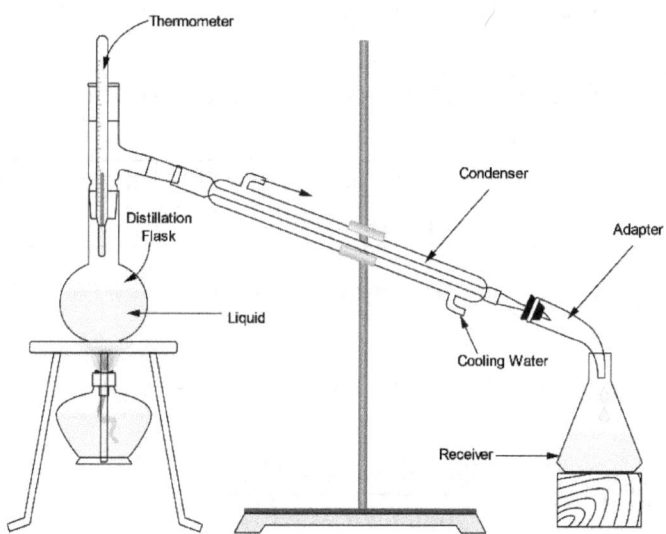

Figure 8.1: Apparatus for Azeotropic distillation

OBSERVATIONS AND CALCULATIONS

Boiling point of alcohol from alcohol-water-glycerin mixture =
Volume of alcohol distilled =

Specific gravity of distilled alcohol =

Percent recovery of alcohol = $\dfrac{\text{volume collected}}{\text{volume used}}$ x 100 =

REPORT:

Strength of alcohol obtained by distillation =

Azeotropic distillation is: **suitable/unsuitable**

Example:

Calculate per cent of alcohol with the data given below:

Sl.No.	Particulars	Weights, g
1	Weight of empty specific gravity bottle, W_1	1.887
2	Weight of empty specific gravity bottle + water, W_2	39.884
3	Weight of empty specific gravity bottle + alcohol, W_4 g	39.201

Weight of water, $W_3 = (W_2 - W_1) = 23.997$ g

Weight of alcohol = $W_5 = (W_4 - W_1) = 23.314$ g

Density of water = $\dfrac{\text{weight of water x 0.980}}{\text{volume of water}}$

$= \dfrac{23.997 \times 0.980}{25} = 0.9407$ g/ml

Density of alcohol = $\dfrac{\text{weight of alcohol}}{\text{weight of water}}$ x Density of water

$$= \frac{23.314}{23.997} \times 0.9407 = 0.9139$$

This value matches with 90.12% of alcohol of the list. Therefore, the alcohol distilled is of 90.12% pure.

QUESTION BANK

1. What is meant by constant boiling mixture? Give one example.
2. Explain the separation of an azeotropic mixture with a suitable example.
3. What do you mean by minimum boiling point and maximum boiling point azeotropic solutions? Draw relevant graphs.
4. Explain the influence of benzene on the azeotropic mixture of ethyl alcohol and water during distillation.
5. Define azeotropic distillation.
6. Write the principle involved in the preparation of absolute alcohol.
7. Describe the principle involved in the azeotropic distillation with a suitable example.

Specific gravity	% ethyl alcohol	Specific gravity	% ethyl alcohol	Specific gravity	% ethyl alcohol
0.9695	96.88	0.9800	60.60	0.9905	26.68
0.9700	95.20	0.9805	58.88	0.9910	25.16
0.9705	93.52	0.9810	57.20	0.9915	23.64
0.9710	91.84	0.9815	55.52	0.9920	22.16
0.9715	90.12	0.9820	53.84	0.9925	20.68
0.9720	88.44	0.9825	52.16	0.9930	19.24
0.9725	86.72	0.9830	50.52	0.9935	17.80
0.9730	85.00	0.9835	48.88	0.9940	16.36
0.9735	83.28	0.9840	47.24	0.9945	14.96
0.9740	81.52	0.9845	45.64	0.9950	13.56
0.9745	79.80	0.9850	44.00	0.9955	12.16
0.9750	78.00	0.9855	42.40	0.9960	10.80
0.9755	76.24	0.9860	40.84	0.9965	9.40
0.9760	74.48	0.9865	39.24	0.9970	8.04
0.9765	72.72	0.9870	37.64	0.9975	6.68
0.9770	70.96	0.9875	36.04	0.9980	5.36
0.9775	69.20	0.9880	34.44	0.9985	4.00
0.9780	67.48	0.9885	32.88	0.9990	2.64
0.9785	65.76	0.9890	31.32	0.9-995	1.32
0.9790	64.00	0.9895	29.76	1.0000	0.00
0.9795	62.32	0.9900	28.20		

SECTION-V
DRYING

Expt-9: Determination of Rate of Drying, Free Moisture Content and Bound Moisture Content

AIM:

To determine the rate of drying for the given sample.

REQUIREMENT:

Petri dish, Hot air oven, Thermometer, Spatula, $CaCO_3$, Weighing balance, and weights

THEORY:

Drying is a *unit operation.* It is a process of removal of trace amount of elements (moisture) from a liquid (or) gas (or) solid (or) semi-solid, at temperature lower than boiling point of materials.

Heat and mass transfers are involved in this process. Drying is a process, which ensures the stability of the product. Tray dryer is a static bed dryer and mechanism of heat transfer is "Convection". It is used for drying of crude drugs, granules etc.

APPLICATIONS

1. In the manufacture of bulk drugs, drying is the final stage of processing. Example is dried Aluminium Hydroxide Gel.
2. Drying is necessary in order to avoid deterioration, for example, crude drugs of animal and vegetable origin.
3. Granules are dried to improve the fluidity and compression characteristics.
4. Drying of viscous and sticky materials modifies the flow characteristics.
5. Removal of moisture makes the material light in weight and reduces the bulk.

Based on Moisture content present in a sample, several terms are expressed:

Equilibrium moisture content (EMC) is the amount of water present in the solid that exerts a vapour pressure equal to the vapour pressure of the atmosphere surrounding it.

Free moisture content (FMC) is defined as the amount of water that is free to evaporate from the solid surface.

FMC = Total water content – Equilibrium moisture content

PRINCIPLE:

The experimental data obtained in an investigation of the effect of external conditions on the drying of a solid by air are usually the moisture content of the solid as a function of time under *constant drying conditions*. The term constant drying conditions means that the air velocity, temperature, humidity, and pressure are maintained constant and that the outlet air conditions are substantially the same as those at the inlet.

The behavior of drying of solids is explained by drying curve. The time required for drying is a batch weight of material in dryer can be estimated with the help of *"Drying Curve"*. The drying rate curve may be divided into a **Constant Rate Period**, such as the portion 'AB' in the following diagram, and the **Falling—Rate Period** 'BD'. The free moisture content at point 'B' is called the **Critical Moisture Content**. If the desired moisture content is larger than the critical moisture content, only the constant rate period will occur.

The rate of drying can be calculated as the ratio of the moisture lost per Sq. cm. per given time. The rate of drying is a standard parameter for several drugs, and can be determined by calculating the amount of water, it need to take (or) to makeup slurry and calculated by a series of drying under consecutive time intervals. The rate of drying can be calculated by the formula.

$$\text{Rate of Drying} = (W_n - W_{n+1}) / \Delta t.A$$

Where,

A = Area of the plate expose to drying

W_n = Weight of glass dish + sample slurry

W_{n+1} = Weight of glass dish + sample slurry after time "t".

Pharmaceutical Engineering Experimental Lab Manual-I (Unit Operations)

Determine the diameter of the given glass dish and calculate the area $(A = \pi r^2)$, Δt-time interval.

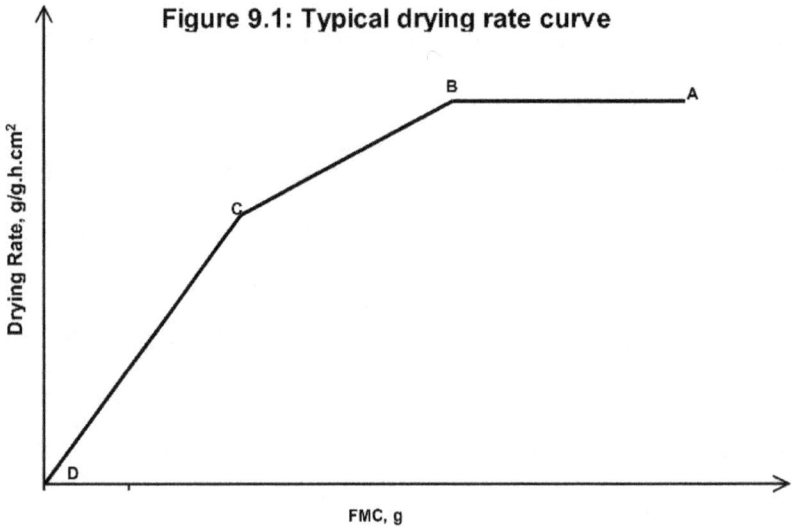

Figure 9.1: Typical drying rate curve

PROCEDURE:

1. Take a clean Petri dish without lid and determine its weight and area of the petri dish, as "W_1", "A" respectively.
2. Take the given powder sample (10 gm. of $CaCO_3$) and fill the petri dish and determine its weight 'W_2'.
3. Make the powder into slurry in the petri dish with the water, and add little more in it, so that a thin layer of water forms above. Let its weight be 'W_3' gm.
4. Now, the petri dish containing slurry is kept in drier (Hot Air Oven) at 70 °C.

5. Continue drying and determine the weight of the sample at every 15 min. interval of time. The weight is recorded in column 3 of the **Table 9.1**.
6. Again, the steel plate containing slurry is placed in the dryer. (Steel plate should be immediately placed back into the dryer, otherwise temperature decreases enormously and results will be erroneous).
7. Steps 5 and 6 are repeated until constant weight is obtained.
8. The rate of drying is calculated.
9. A graph is plotted by taking **Free Moisture Content** (weight of water, column 5) on *x-axis* and **Rate of Drying** (column 9) on *y-axis*. (A model graph is shown in **Figure 9.1**).

OBSERVATIONS AND CALCULATIONS

Weight of empty Petri dish, $w_1 =$

Weight of Petri dish + sample slurry, $w_2 =$

Weight of the sample slurry, $w_3 = w_2 - w_1 =$

For example, 45 g of sample slurry contains 10 g of calcium carbonate w_3 g of sample slurry contains? g of calcium carbonate

$$\frac{15 \times w_3}{45} = w_4 \text{ g of calcium carbonate}$$

Weight of Total Water Content (TWC), $w_5 = (w_3 - w_4) =$ _____

Diameter of Petri dish, $d =$ _____ cm

Radius of Petri dish, $r = (d/2) =$ _____ cm

Area of Petri dish, $A = \pi r^2 =$ _____ cm^2

Moisture content removed from the sample = w_2 - Last weight of steel plate taken with sample + water (if any)

REPORT

Drying rate curve is plotted by taking FMC on *x-axis* and rate of drying on *y-axis*.

Total Moisture Content removed from calcium carbonate slurry = _____ g

Example:

Calculate the rate of drying of a given sample.

The data are given below:

Weight of the Petri dish, $w_1 = 28.9$ g

Weight of Petri dish + sample + water, $w_2 = 62.6$ g

Weight of sample taken, $w_4 = 17.3$ g

Weight of water present in the slurry = 16.4 g

After 15 minutes, weight of Petri dish + sample + water = 61.6 g

After 30 minutes, weight of Petri dish + sample + water = 60.6 g

Surface area of the slurry exposed to hot air (Petri dish) = 70.85 cm^2

Section-V Expt-9: Rate of Drying

Solution:

At 15 minutes:

Weight of sample + Weight of water = 61.6 - 28.9 = 32.7 g

Weight of water, w_4 = 32.7 - 17.3 = 15.4 g.

Weight of water removed = Total Water Content - Weight of water left in the sample

= 16.4 - 15.4 = 1.0 g.

At 15 minutes time:

Weight of water lost per gram of dry powder = 1.0/17.3 = 0.0578 g/g

At 30 minutes:

Weight of sample + Weight of water = 60.6 - 28.9 = 31.7 g

Weight of water, w_4 = 31.7 - 17.3 = 14.4 g.

Weight of water removed = Total Water Content - Weight of water left in the sample

= 16.4 - 14.4 = 2.0 g.

At 30 minutes time:

Weight of water lost per gram of dry powder = 2.0/17.3 = 0.1156 g/g

Drying in the time interval = 0.1156 - 0.0578 = 0.0578 g/g

Rate of drying of substance per g per hr = $\dfrac{0.0578 \times 60}{15}$ = 0.2312 g/g.h

Rate of drying of substance per g per hr per cm^2 = $\dfrac{0.2312}{70.85}$ = 0.00326 g/g.h.cm^2

Solution:

At 15 minutes:

Weight of sample + Weight of water = 61.6-28.9 = 32.7 g

Weight of water, w_4 = 32.7 – 17.3 = 15.4 g.

Weight of water removed = Total Water Content – Weight of water left in the sample

= 16.4 – 15.4 = 1.0 g.

At 15 minutes time:

Weight of water lost per gram of dry powder = 1.0/17.3 = 0.0578 g/g

At 30 minutes:

Weight of sample + Weight of water = 60.6-28.9 = 31.7 g

Weight of water, w_4 = 31.7 – 17.3 = 14.4 g.

Weight of water removed = Total Water Content – Weight of water left in the sample

= 16.4 – 14.4 = 2.0 g.

At 30 minutes time:

Weight of water lost per gram of dry powder = 2.0/17.3 = 0.1156 g/g

Drying in the time interval = 0.1156 – 0.0578 = 0.0578 g/g

Section-V   Expt-9: Rate of Drying

Rate of drying of substance per g per hr = $\dfrac{0.0578 \times 60}{15}$ = 0.2312 g/g.h

Rate of drying of substance per g per hr per cm² = $\dfrac{0.2312}{70.85}$ = 0.00326 g/g.h.cm²

Table 9.1: Drying Rate of Calcium Carbonate

Sl. No.	Drying time, min	Weight of Petri dish + wt. of calcium carbonate + wt. of water, g	Weight of calcium carbonate + wt. of water, g	Free moisture content, g	Weight of water remained (present)/gram of dry powder, g/g
			(3) - w_1	(4) – w_4	(5)/w_4,
(1)	(2)	(3)	(4)	(5)	(6)
1	0				
2	15				
3	30				
4	45				
5	60				
6	75				
7	90				
8	105				
9	120				

Drying in the time interval, g/g.min	Rate of drying per hour; g/g.h	Rate of drying per hour per gram per surface area exposed, g/g.h.cm^2
$6_{(n-1)} - 6_{(n)}$ / $(2)_n - (2)_{n-1}$	(7) x 60	(8) / A
(7)	(8)	(9)

QUESTION BANK:

1. Define drying. How is it difference between from evaporation and distillation?
2. Enumerate pharmaceutical applications of drying.
3. Define the terms: a) Equilibrium moisture content; b) Free moisture content; c) Critical moisture content; d) Bound water; e) Unbound water.
4. Draw a typical labelled drying rate curve.
5. List a few laboratory scale dryers.
6. Describe the mechanisms of drying during constant drying rate period, first falling rate period, and second falling rate period.
7. Describe the principle involved in the drying of a substance with a suitable example.

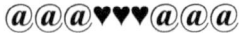

SECTION-VI
FILTRATION

Expt-10: Effect of Factors on Filtration Rate-Materials Related Factors (Effect of Filter Aids on Rate of Filtration)

AIM:

To study the effect of Filter Aids on the rate of filtration and to determine the optimum concentration of filter aid.

REQUIREMENT:

Filter Aids (Bentonite & Talc), Calcium carbonate, Water

PRINCIPLE:

The filter aid is a finely divided solid material, but consisting of hard strong particles that are *masse* incompressible, for sludge's that are difficult to filter. Filter aid forms a surface deposit, which screens out the solids and also for events the plugging of the filter media. The various filter aids are used in the pharmaceutical field, depending on their usage and availability.

Ex: Kieselguhr/diatomaceous earth, asbestos, talc and charcoal etc.

The most important filter aid, widely used is diatomaceous earth or kieselguhr. It consists of siliceous skeletons of very small marine organisms known as 'diatoms.'

THEORY:

Slimy or very fine solids that form a dense impermeable cake quickly plug any filter medium that is fine enough to retain them. Practical filtration of such materials requires that the porosity of the cake be increased to permit passage of the liquor at a reasonable rate, this is done by adding a filter aid.

Filter aid can be used in either of *three* (3) ways:

1. Use *of pre-coat* of filter aid or thin layer of the material lay down on the filter before the sludge proper is pumped to the apparatus. A pre-coat prevents the colloidal particles of the sludge from becoming so enlarged in the filter cloth that, the resistance of the end of filtration.

2. Using filter aid is the incorporation of a certain percentage of the material with the sludge before sending it to the press. The presence of the filter aid increases the porosity of the sludge, decease its compressibility, and reduces the resistance of the cake during filtration.

3. Using filter aid is the use of special *pre-coat. filter*. This is essentially a rotary-drum vacuum filter. Slurry of filter aid only is fed to the filter until a layer of pre-coat 2" (inch) or thicker has been laid down. Then sludge to be filtered is fed. The doctor knife is so positioned that it peels off the sludge and an extremely thin layer of the pre-coat. Filtration is then interrupted, a new thick layer of pre-coat deposited, and

filtration continued. This method is used for slimy or gelatinous precipitates that can never be built up to a cake but must be removed when the filter has on it a very thin layer of the precipitate.

The object of the filter aid is to prevent the medium from becoming blocked and to form an open porous cake. Hence, reduce the resistance to flow of filtering solution.

PROCEDURE:

1. Weigh accurately 5 gm of Calcium Carbonate, transfer to graduated conical flask and add water to dissolve Calcium carbonate and make up volume up to 100 ml.
2. Prepare solutions like step No: 1 for about 6 numbers in different conical flasks.
3. Then add Bentonite in the concentrations of 0.1 %, 0.2 %, 0.3%, 0.4% and 0.5% to the above five (5) solutions.
4. Number the conical flasks with numerical numbers like 1, 2, 3, 4, 5 & 6.
5. Now, pass the first sample (Control) [i.e., 0.0% bentonite in 5% calcium carbonate] marked as No: 1 through a selected filter paper and note down time taken for filtration.
6. Similarly, repeat the entire experiment for the other remaining solutions and determine time required for filtration and record them in the observation by using the following table.

Pharmaceutical Engineering Experimental Lab Manual-I (Unit Operations)

Determination of Optimum Concentration:

To know the optimum concentration of filtration aid, draw a graph by taking filter aid on X-axis and rate filtration on Y- axis.

As the concentration of filter aid is increased, rate of filtration also increases but the point reaches where further additions of filter aid decreases the rate of filtration. The concentration at this change is optimum concentration of filter aid.

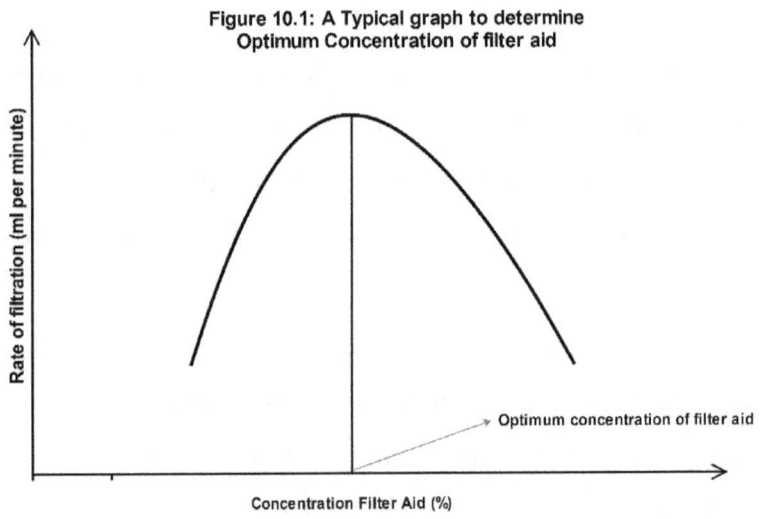

Figure 10.1: A Typical graph to determine Optimum Concentration of filter aid

OBSERVATIONS AND CALCULATIONS:

S. No	Volume of 5% Calcium carbonate	Concentration of filter aid (%)	Time taken for filtration (minutes)	Rate of filtration (ml per minute)
1	100 ml	0.0		
2	100 ml	0.1		
3	100 ml	0.2		
4	100 ml	0.3		
5	100 ml	0.4		
6	100 ml	0.5		

Section-VI   Expt-10: Filtration Rate-Materials related Factors

REPORT:

The Optimum concertation of filter aid (Bentonite/ Kieselguhr / Talc) was found to be _____%

Example:

For the filtration of a 5 % calcium carbonate suspension, the volume of filtrate collected in 20 min is 142.5 ml. Calculate the rate of filtration in m^3/s.

Solution:

Volume of filtrate collected = 142.5 ml; Time of filtration = 20 minutes.

Rate of filtration (ml/min) = 142.5/ 20 = 7.125 ml/ min.

Rate of filtration (m^3/s) = 7.125 x 10^{-6} / 60 = 0.01188 x 10^{-6} m^3/s

QUESTION BANK

1. Explain the mechanisms of surface filtration.
2. What happens to the rate of filtration, when concentration of suspended particles is increased? Justify.
3. How is filtration different from clarification?
4. Describe four applications of filtration.
5. List the material related factors influencing the filtration.

@@@♥♥@@@

Expt-11: Effect of Factors on Filtration Rate-Process Related Factors

AIM:
To study the effect of various factors on the rate of filtration.

REQUIREMENTS
Filter paper, vacuum pump, Buchner funnel, stop clock

PRINCIPLE:
Filtration is a process whereby solid particles present in a suspension are separated from the liquid or gas employing a porous medium, which retains the solid but allows the fluid to pass through. The volume of the filtrate obtained through the filter paper per unit time is called Rate of filtration. The rate of filtration can be given by mathematical equation.

$$dv/dt = K.A.\Delta P/ \mu.I \text{-----------------------Darcy's Law}$$

Where; A = Area of filter; ΔP = Pressure drop across the filter medium & cake; μ= Viscosity of filtrate; I = thickness of cake; V =Volume of the filtrate; t = time taken for filtration; K = Constant for the filter medium & filter cake (or) Resistance Procedure

Effect of Thickness of Cake:

Prepare two solutions of calcium carbonate using water as the solvent; the concentrations of the solutions are 5% & 10 % respectively. Filter them and note the time taken for filtration to calculate the rate of filtration & compare them.

Effect of Viscosity:

(using two solutions, one with water and other with mixture of glycerin and water (20:80 ratio) respectively). Prepare two different solutions of 5% $CaCO_3$- using above prepared water & glycerin mixture. Filter them and note the time for filtration to calculate the rate of filtration & compare them.

Effect of Area:

This can be determined by using funnel of large (big) and small areas for the same concentration of the solution (5% $CaCO_3$). Times taken for filtrations are noted, & calculate the rate of filtration and compare them.

Effect of Pressure:

Prepare two solutions of calcium carbonate (5% of each) using water as solvent. Filter one of the solutions through a Buchner funnel, which is connected to a suction pump, and the other one is filtered through without suction pump and note the time taken for filtration, calculate the rate of filtration & compare them.

OBSERVATION AND CALCULATIONS:

1. Effect of Thickness:

Sample: 50 ml of 5% $CaCO_3$ 50 ml of 10% $CaCO_3$

Sample	Time taken for filtration	Vol. of filtrate	Rate of filtration
5% $CaCO_3$			
10% $CaCO_3$			

2. Effect of Viscosity:

Sample: 50 ml of 5% $CaCO_3$

50 ml of 5% $CaCO_3$ [glycerin water mixture (20: 80: glycerin: water)]

Sample	Time taken for filtration	Vol. of filtrate	Rate of filtration
5% $CaCO_3$			
5% $CaCO_3$ with glycerin water mixture			

3. Effect of Area of the Funnel:

Sample: 50 ml of 5% $CaCO_3$

Sample	Time taken for filtration	Vol. of filtrate	Rate of filtration
5% $CaCO_3$ filter in small funnel			
5% $CaCO_3$ filter in big funnel			

4. Effect of Pressure:

Sample: 50 ml of 5% CaCO$_3$ [glycerin water mixture (20: 80: glycerin: water)]

Sample	Time taken for filtration	Vol. of filtrate	Rate of filtration
5% CaCO$_3$ filter with Pressure			
5% CaCO$_3$ filter without Pressure			

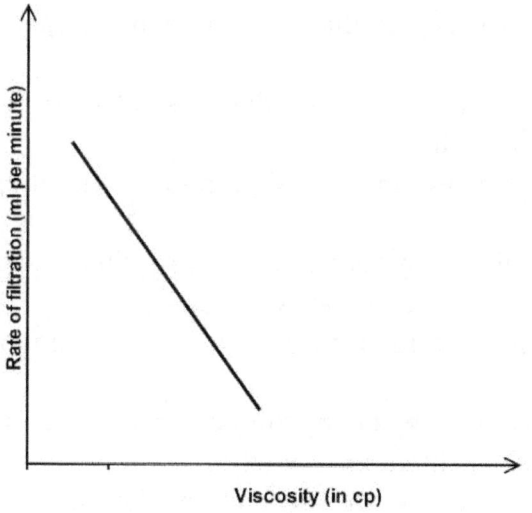

Figure 11.1: A graph between Rate of filtration Vs Viscosity

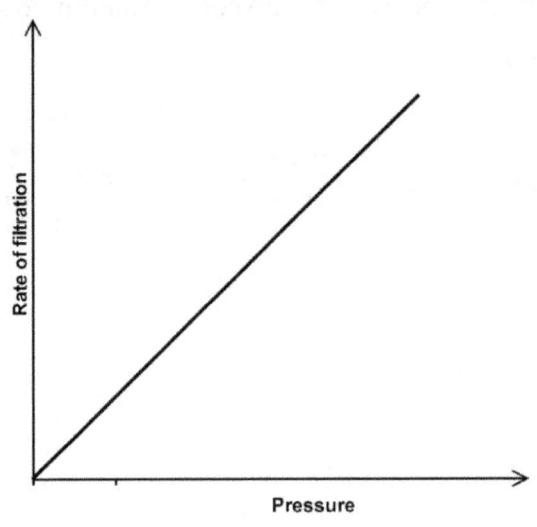

Figure 11.2: A graph, between Rate of filtration Vs Pressure

REPORT:

1. With the increase in thickness, rate of filtration increases/ decreases.
   A Graph is plotted by taking thickness of filter medium on x-axis and rate of filtration on y-axis.
2. With the increase in viscosity, rate of filtration increases/ decreases.
   A Graph is plotted by taking viscosity of filter medium on x-axis and rate of filtration on y-axis.
3. With the increase in surface area, rate of filtration increases/ decreases.
   A Graph is plotted by taking Surface area of filter medium on x-axis and rate of filtration on y-axis.
4. With the application of vaccum, rate of filtration increases/ decreases.
   A bar graph is plotted by taking atmospheric pressure on x-axis and rate of filtration on y-axis.

QUESTION BANK:

1. What are the factors influencing the rate of filtration?
2. Differentiate between pressure filtration and vaccum filtration.

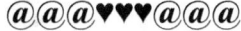

SECTION-VII
HUMIDITY

Expt-12: Determination of Humidity-Psychometric Method

AIM:

To determine the humidity and relative humidity of the ambient environment using psychrometer.

THEORY

Humidity is defined as the ratio of mass of water present in the air to the mass of dry air. Humidity has the units of kg/kg. The concentration of water vapour in a gas is called the humidity of gas. Humidity is also known as humidity ratio or relative humidity, which is expressed as percentage. Relative humidity is defined as the ratio of actual humidity to the saturation humidity at a temperature. Wet bulb and dry bulb temperatures are important for the determination of humidity. Dry bulb temperature is the temperature of the moist air when it is measured at rest, which is not affected by the moisture content of the air or by radiation. Wet bulb temperature is the dynamic equilibrium temperature attained by a water surface, when exposed to air under adiabatic conditions. The other methods used for measuring the humidity are gravimetric method and dew point method, hygrometer (mechanical and electric). Since heat transfer and mass transfer are observed in the wet bulb temperature, their coefficients are important and are influenced by many factors. The wet bulb temperature depends upon the humidity and temperature of air.

SLING PSYCHROMETER:

Sling psychrometer consists of two similar thermometers that are fixed to a metal frame (Figure). The bulb of one thermometer is kept open to the ambient conditions. This thermometer gives dry bulb temperature. The bulb of second thermometer is kept moist by a wet cotton wick immersed in a water reservoir. This thermometer gives wet bulb temperature. When the sling psychrometer is kept for a while, the wet bulb temperature reaches a minimum and remains constant. The temperatures of two thermometers are noted.

Psychrometric Charts:

Psychrometry is a term used for determining the vapour concentration and carrying capacity of the gas. For engineering calculations, the properties of mixture of air and water vapour are necessary. Humidity charts or psychrometric charts are helpful for this purpose.

Figure 12.1. Sling psychrometer

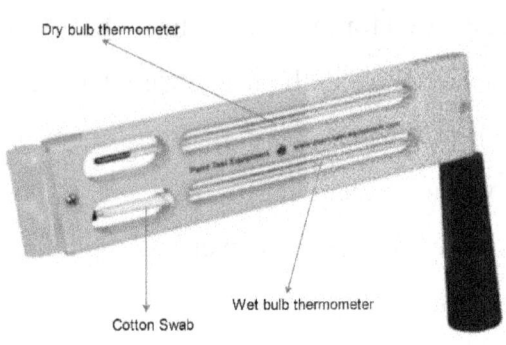

The following parameters are include& in the psychrometric charts.

-Humidity vs. temperature

-Humid heat vs. humidity

-Specific volume vs. temperature

-Adiabatic cooling lines (or constant wet bulb temperature lines)

-Saturation humidity curve

Saturation humidity is absolute humidity at which the partial pressure of water vapour in the air is equal to the vapour pressure of free water at the same temperature. These plots are considered for the determination of existing conditions of environment at constant pressure. Based on these values, the desirable environmental conditions are established by suitable adjustment of the equipment.

APPLICATIONS:

1. The humidity conditions of the air are important for determining operating conditions for drying of substances.
2. Based on humidity needs, condensers, cooling towers, dehumidifier, and air conditioners are designed. Air conditioning is a critical factor in the manufacturing area of dosage forms, tablets, capsules, sterile products etc.

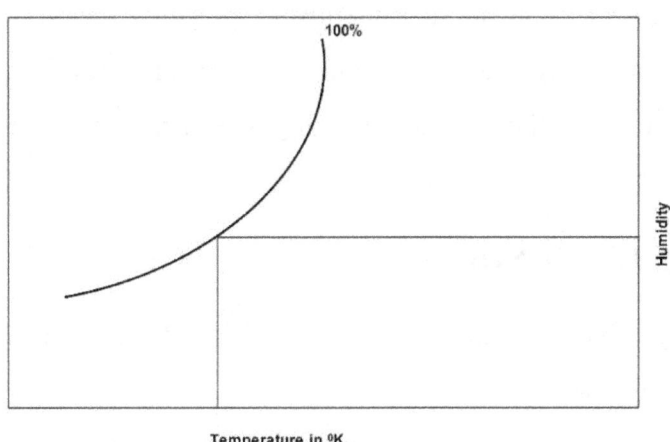

Figure 12.2: Psychrometric chart

LIMITATIONS:

The skill in handling and space for keeping the sling psychrometer are the limitations. The assumption that the wet bulb temperature is equal to the adiabatic saturation temperature does not hold true, for non-aqueous systems.

PRINCIPLE

Sling thermometer gives wet bulb and dry bulb temperatures. The wet bulb temperature is a function of temperature and humidity of air used for evaporation. The differences between the wet bulb and dry bulb temperatures are used for calculating the per cent relative humidity and humidity of air.

$$\text{Percent Relative Humidity} = \frac{\text{Humidity of air}}{\text{Humidity of saturated air}}$$

The intersection point is identified at which the saturated curve crosses the wet bulb temperature. From this point, the horizontal line towards the y-axis (humidity scale) is drawn and humidity values are noted.

REQUIREMENTS

Sling Psychrometer containing Wet Bulb and Dry Bulb thermometers

PROCEDURE

Laboratory Conditions—Humidity

1. The sling psychrometer is taken and verified for the dry bulb thermometer, which is exposed to open air. The wet bulb thermometer is verified for its cloth sack dipping in the water present in the plastic container.
2. The sling psychrometer is whirled in the air of laboratory.
3. The dry bulb and wet bulb temperatures are noted at 5 minute intervals. Once the temperatures remained constant, these are

considered as dry bulb and wet bulb temperatures for calculations.

4. The humidity and relative humidity are determined using humidity charts.

Open Air of the College Building-Humidity

Repeat the steps 2 to 4 as mentioned above.

OBSERVATIONS AND CALCULATIONS

Table 12.1: Dry bulb and Wet bulb temperatures at different locations:

Sl.No	Name of the location	Average dry bulb temperature		Average wet bulb temperature		Humidity	Percent relative humidity
		°C	°F	°C	°F		
1.							
2.							
		Average Humidity =					

REPORT

Humidity of the air =

Per cent relative humidity =

Example:

The wet bulb and dry bulb temperatures of air at atmospheric pressure are 26°C and 32°C, respectively. Calculate the humidity and per cent relative humidity.

Solution:

HUMIDITY:

The wet bulb temperature is 26°C or 26±273.12 = 299.12 K. The wet bulb temperature, the corresponding *Adiabatic Cooling Line* is identified. Along this line, proceeded to the 100% humidity (**Saturated Curve**). The intersect point is identified and the coordinates (x, y) are noted.

From the psychrometric chart, this point is 299 K, 0.022 kg/kg).
The y coordinate, i.e., 0.022 kg/kg, is the humidity.

PER CENT RELATIVE HUMIDITY:

From the above intersect point, move horizontally moves up to dry bulb temperature, 32°C or 32 ± 273.12 = 305.12 K or 305 K. The intersect point on the vertical line is identified. The curve that passes through this intersect represents the per cent humidity. For the above data, the per cent relative humidity is 70% RH.

Alternatively, dry bulb temperature is considered on x-axis. From this point, moved vertically up to 100% humidity (saturation curve) and intersect point is identified. The coordinates of the intersect point are obtained.

From psychrometric chart, the coordinates are 305, 0.031.

The saturation humidity is 0.031.

$$\text{Per cent relative humidity} = \frac{\text{Humidity of air}}{\text{Humidity of saturated air}} \times 100 = 71\%$$

QUESTION BANK

1. What is the difference between humidity and relative humidity with respect to air?
2. Define the terms, 'specific humidity' and 'relative humidity'?
3. Define various expressions of humidity.
4. List different types of psychrometric parameters.
5. Explain the applications of humidity.
6. Describe the principle involved in the determination of humidity using sling psychrometer.
7. Describe the principle involved in the attainment of low temperature by wet bulb compared to dry bulb temperature.

Expt-13: Determination of Humidity-Dew Point Method

AIM:

To determine the humidity of the air by dew point method.

THEORY

Humidity of the environment is an important factor that is routinely monitored and maintained in the production areas of various unit dosage forms, such as tablets, capsules (hard gelatin and soft gelatin), and sterile products.

PRINCIPLE

Dew point is defined as the temperature to which a mixture of air-water vapour must be cooled (at constant humidity) to become saturated (i.e., to be in equilibrium with liquid).

Formation of mist and disappearance of mist are considered and dew point is determined/Dew point temperature is noted on the temperature axis (x-axis) and moved vertically on the psychrometric chart. The intersect point at saturated curve (100%) is identified. The coordinates of the point (temperature, K, humidity) are noted. The y-axis point is the humidity of air. These values are substituted in the equation.

Percent Relative Humidity $= \dfrac{\text{Humidity of air}}{\text{Humidity of saturated air}} \times 100$

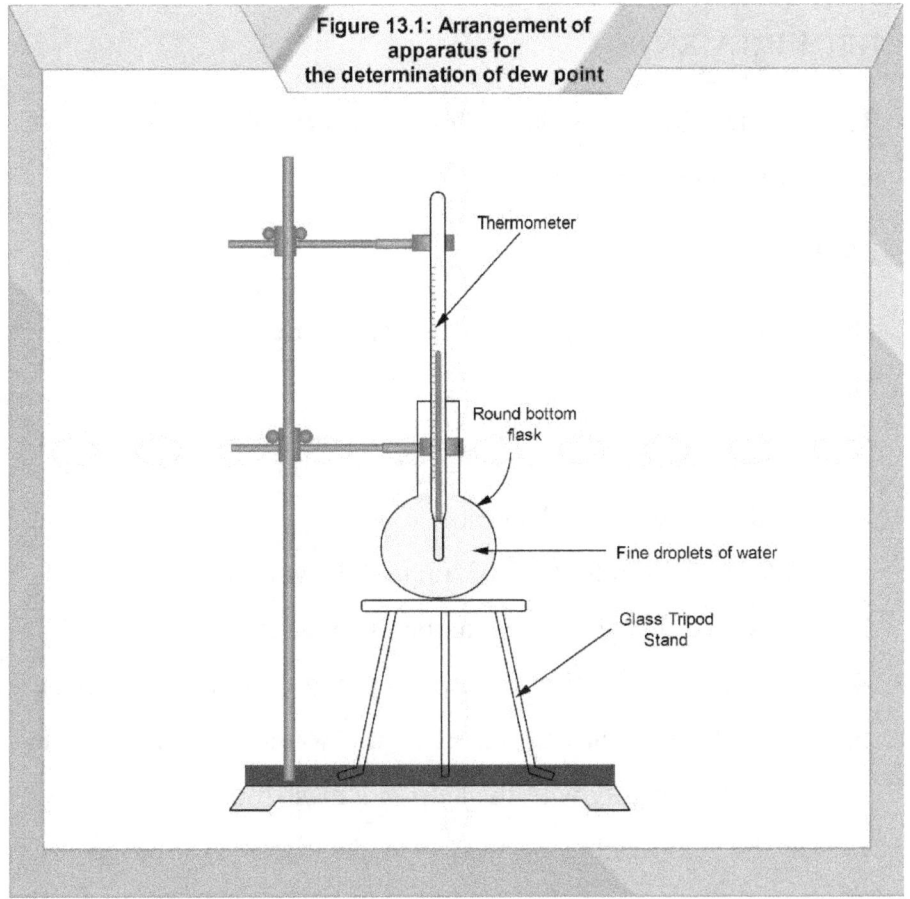

Figure 13.1: Arrangement of apparatus for the determination of dew point

Percent Relative Humidity can be directly read from the psychrometric chart.

The cooled and polished disk is placed in a vessel. The vessel is cooled gradually. At a particular temperature, the mist begins to form and this temperature is noted. It is the dew point. Alternatively, dew point can be determined using a round bottom flask. The arrangement of apparatus is shown in **Figure 13.1**.

REQUIREMENTS

Round bottom long neck flask, 100 ml; water; Thermometer, 110°C; ice; Glass tripod stand.

PROCEDURE

The assembly of apparatus for determining dew point is shown in **Figure**.

1. A round bottom long neck flask (100 ml) is thoroughly cleaned and dried the external surface.
2. Water is filled into the flask up to $2/3^{rd}$ volume.
3. The above flask is kept on a glass tripod stand.
4. A thermometer (110°C) is dipped in the water (**Figure 13.1**).
5. Crushed ice is slowly added to the water (in the flask) and stirred thoroughly with the help of a glass rod.
6. As the temperature of water (in the flask) is lowered, mist begins to form on the outer bottom surface of the flask. At this point, the temperature is noted. This is the dew point (temperature).
7. In psychrometric chart, from the temperature (x-axis) moved vertically up until the saturation curve and identified the intersecting point. The coordinates of the (temperature, humidity) intersecting point are noted. The y coordinate is the humidity.

OBSERVATIONS AND CALCULATIONS

Trials	Dew point, °C		Humidity
	Mist appearance	Average value	
I			
II			

From humidity chart, humidity of saturated air dew point = _____ kg water/kg dry air

$$\text{Percent Relative Humidity} = \frac{\text{Humidity of air}}{\text{Humidity of saturated air}} \times 100$$

REPORT

Humidity of the air =

Per cent relative humidity of air =

Example:

The dew point of air is identified as 17°C. Calculate the humidity of the air.

Solution:

The dew point of the air is 17°C or 17 + 273.12 K or 290 K. This temperature is identified on x-axis. From this point, moved vertically up to 100% RH (saturated humidity) curve. The intersect point on this curve is identified and coordinates are noted. From the psychrometric chart, the coordinate of the intersect is (290 K, 0.014 kg/kg). The y coordinate is the humidity, i.e., 0.014.

QUESTION BANK

1. Explain the principle involved in the determination of humidity by dew point method.
2. Define dew point. How is it identified experimentally?

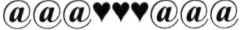

SECTION-VIII
SIZE REDUCTION & SEPARATION

Expt-14: Determination of Efficiency of Size Reduction of a Mixer and A Ball Mill

AIM:

To compare the efficiency of size reduction of a mixer and a ball

REQUIREMENTS:

Ball mill, Mixer/Blender, Dill fruits, Coriander fruits, sieves # 10, 22, 44, 80, 100 & 120 and sieve shaker.

OBJECTIVES:

The objectives of the size reduction are to get improved dissolution rate, improved rate of absorption, effective extraction of drugs, effective drying, improved physical stability, uniform flow and content uniformity, etc.

THEORY:

Size reduction is the process of reducing substances to small particles. This unit operation is also commonly known as *comminution* or *diminution* or *grinding* or *pulverization* and is extensively used in pharmaceutical operations both in the laboratory and on the industrial scale. Size reduction increases surface area of the material and the greater the surface area of the material the higher the rate of dissolution of the material in a suitable solvent. Normally size reduction may be achieved by two methods, namely *precipitation* or *mechanical* process.

There are four types of modes of stress applied in size reduction,

    i. Cutting, Ex: Cutter mill
    ii. Compression, Ex: Roller mill
    iii. Impact, Ex: Hammer mill
    iv. Attrition, Ex: Fluid energy mill

The ball mill consists of a horizontally rotating hallow vessel of cylindrical shape with the length slightly greater than its diameter. The mill is partially filled with balls of steel or pebbles. The load of balls in a ball mill is normally such that when the mill is stopped, the balls occupy about one half the volume of the mill. The void fraction in the mass of balls, when at rest, is typically 0.40. The grinding may be done with dry solids, but more commonly the feed is a suspension of the particles in water, increasing both the capacity and the efficiency of the mill.

PRINCIPLE:

The ball mill works on the principle of *Impact* and *Attrition* between the rapidly moving balls and the powder material. both enclosed a hallow cylinder. At low speeds, the balls roll over each other and attrition (rubbing action) will be the predominant mode of action. Thus, in the ball mill, impact or attrition or both are responsible for the size reduction.

In the cutter mill, size reduction involves successive cutting or shearing the feed material with the help of sharp knives or blades. This is used to obtain a coarse degree of size reduction of soft materials. The commonest application is the treatment of drugs such as roots, peels or foods, and prior to extraction.

PROCEDURE:

1. Take equally weighed (5 gm. each) amounts of *CORIANDER* and *DILL* fruits.

2. Divide into two successive portions (each of 2.5 gm) in ball mill and Mixer/Blender respectively.

3. Both are operated for 15 & 30 min. The powdered drug is put in a set of sieves (#10, 22, 44, 80, 100 & 120) and undergone for shaking with the help of sieve shaker for about 10 min.

4. The amount retained on each mesh is noted by weighing of individual powder.

5. The same process is repeated for Dill fruits and amount retained on each sieve is noted.

6. Finally find out the percentage amount retained on each sieve and give report.

7. Observation After 15 min

Table 14.1: Coriander obtained from MIXER/BLENDER.

S. No.	Sieve No.	Amt. Retained (in gms)	Percentage retained
1	10		
2	77		
3	44		
4	80		
5	100		
6	120		

Table 14.2 Coriander obtained from BALL MILL.

S. No.	Sieve No.	Amt. Retained (in gms)	Percentage retained
1	10		
2	22		
3	44		
4	80		
5	100		
6	120		

Table 14.3 Dill obtained from MIXER/BLENDER.

S. No.	Sieve No.	Amt. Retained (in gms)	Percentage retained
1	10		
2	22		
3	44		
4	80		
5	100		
6	120		

Table 14.4: Dill obtained from BALL MILL.

S. No.	Sieve No.	Amt. Retained (in gms)	Percentage retained
1	10		
2	22		
3	44		
4	80		
5	100		
6	120		

After 30 min:

Table 14.5 Coriander obtained from MIXER/BLENDER.

S. No.	Sieve No.	Amt. Retained (in gms)	Percentage retained
1	10		
2	22		
3	44		
4	80		
5	100		
6	120		

Table 14.6 Coriander obtained from BALL MILL.

S. No.	Sieve No.	Amt. Retained (in gms)	Percentage retained
1	10		
2	22		
3	44		
4	80		
5	100		
6	120		

Table 14.7 Dill obtained from MIXER/BLENDER.

S. No.	Sieve No.	Amt. Retained (in gms)	Percentage retained
1	10		
2	22		
3	44		
4	80		
5	100		
6	120		

Table 14.8 Dill obtained from BALL MILL.

S. No.	Sieve No.	Amt. Retained (in gms)	Percentage retained
1	10		
2	22		
3	44		
4	80		
	100		
6	120		

Pharmaceutical Engineering Experimental Lab Manual-I (Unit Operations)

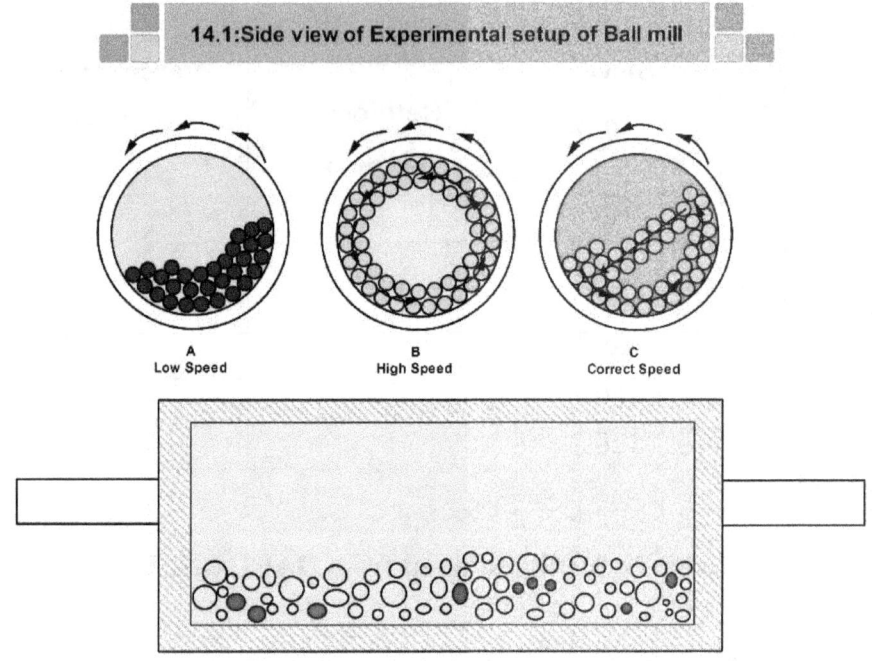

14.1: Side view of Experimental setup of Ball mill

A — Low Speed
B — High Speed
C — Correct Speed

@@@♥♥@@@

SECTION-IX
MIXING

Expt-15: Mixing Index of a Blender - Calcium Carbonate and Talc

AIM:

To determine the mixing index for the blending of calcium carbonate and talc in a blender.

THEORY

Mixing is defined as a process that tends to result in a randomization of dissimilar particles within a system.

The term *mix* means to put together in one mass or assemblage with more or less thorough diffusion of the constituents among one another. The term *blending* means to mix smoothly and inseparably together. During blending, a minimum energy is imparted to the bed. These terms are commonly used interchangeably in the industry.

In the solid-solid mixing operations four steps are involved. These are:

1. Expansion of the bed of solids.

2. Application of three-dimensional shear forces to the powder bed.
3. Long term mixing to obtain true randomization of particles.
4. Maintaining randomization (no segregation after mixing).

When dry materials are loaded into a mixer, they form a static bed. This bed expands sufficiently when mixing is initiated. Therefore, there should be enough void space in the mixer after it is charged with the ingredients. The shear force produces movement of particles. The stress induces the movement of particles in three directions. This turbulent movement of particles can bring about randomization. If the forces are inadequate, particle agglomerates move together leading to poor mixing.

Initially the rate of mixing is rapid, later the rate decreases. Since the rate process follows first order (asymptotic), perfect mixing is not attainable, i.e., it takes infinite time. Empirically the best mixing time would be 30 to 35 minutes. Once the desired mixture is achieved, the process should be stopped. Once the mixing is stopped, the blend exists in static equilibrium. Subsequent handling of the mixture should be so as not to disturb the static equilibrium.

The equipment used for mixing of solids are cylindrical blender, cube blender, V-cone blender, double cone blender, ribbon blender, sigma blade mixer, planetary mixer, barrel type mixer and zigzag mixer. Cylindrical blender used for mixing of solids is shown in **Figure 15.1.**

Figure 15.1. Cylindrical blender with baffles

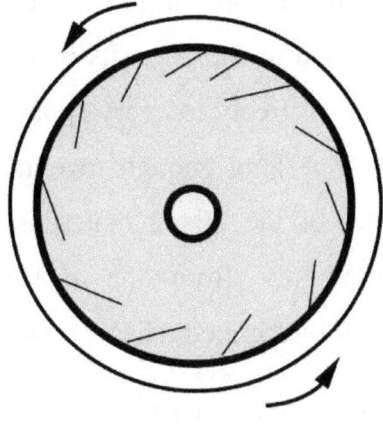

2 -D diagram

APPLICATIONS:

Mixing is one of the most widely used unit operation in the pharmaceutical industries. It is used as an intermediate step or used as final step or used alone in the manufacture of dosage formulations.

a) Powders are mixed with the liquid during preparation of wet granules for the production of tablets and capsules.

b) Powders are mixed in dry condition to prepare them for direct compression.

c) For the manufacture of dry syrups and compound powders dry blending is important.

d) Potent drugs are supplied by mixing with adjuvants.

PRINCIPLE

Mixing of calcium carbonate and talc is studied using cylindrical blender. Blender is allowed to rotate on its own axis. During this process, the particles move freely to every spot of the equipment. Time of mixing should be long enough to obtain an acceptable randomization. Samples of the mixed materials are collected at different intervals randomly from the different spots. The components are analysed by the method acid-base titration.

Amount of calcium carbonate is determined by treating the sample with known excess of hydrochloric acid. Unreacted hydrochloric acid solution can be determined by back titrating against sodium hydroxide solution using phenolphthalein as indicator.

Mixing index refers to the degree of uniformity achieved during mixing. It is calculated by a statistical procedure. Mixing index is determined using the following formula:

$$M_s = \frac{\Sigma (y-\bar{y})^2}{n(1-\bar{y})\bar{y}}$$

Where, M_s = mixing index; n = number of samples; $\bar{y}$ = true average composition of component A in the mixture y = actual composition of component A in a single sample

M_s values are calculated at different time intervals. Based on results, optimum time required for actual mixing is estimated. A graph can be plotted by taking time of mixing on x-axis and mixing index on y-axis.

REQUIREMENTS

Cylindrical blender; 0.1 N hydrochloric acid solution; Stop watch; 0.1 N sodium hydroxide solution; Conical flasks, 250 ml; Phenolphthalein indicator; Pipette, 10 ml; Calcium carbonate; Burette, 50 ml; Talc; Volumetric flask, 100 ml; Oxalic acid; Volumetric flask, 500 ml; Balance; Weight box.

Procedure

1. 5 g of calcium carbonate and 5.0 g of talc are weighed
2. These two powders are placed in a cylindrical blender.
3. The blender is allowed to rotate on its own axis for 10 minutes at 25 revolutions per minute.
4. The samples (500 mg) are drawn from three different places of the blender and placed in three different conical flasks. Labelled them as 1A, 1B, and 1C.
5. The blender is again allowed to rotate for another 10 minutes.
6. Again, three samples are drawn in a similar way as mentioned in step 4. They are transferred into three different conical flasks and labelled them as 2A, 2B, and 2C.
7. Repeat the steps 5 and 6 for another 10 minutes. The samples are labelled as 3A, 3B, and 3C.

8. 30 ml of standard hydrochloric acid solution ($N_3 =$) is placed in each conical flask.
9. The contents of flask are shaken thoroughly to complete the reaction between hydrochloric acid and calcium carbonate.

Unreacted hydrochloric acid is determined by titrating against standard sodium hydroxide solution ($N_2 =$) using phenolphthalein indicator. The readings are recorded in the Table.

The content of calcium carbonate present in each sample is calculated and reported in **Table 15.1**.

The data is substituted in equation (15.1) and the mixing index is calculated for the desired intervals.

A graph is plotted by taking time on *x-axis* and mixing index on *y-axis*.

Weight of the sample taken = 500 mg = 0.5 g

Volume of hydrochloric acid ($N_2 =$) added = 30 ml

Conversion factor *(d)* =

REPORT:

    1. Mixing index after 10 minutes, $M_{10} =$ _____

    2. Mixing index after 20 minutes, $M_{20} =$ _____

    3. Mixing index after 30 minutes, $M_{30} =$ _____

Section-IX Expt-15: Mixing Index-Calcium carbonate and Talc

Example:

Calculate the mixing index for the powder blend of calcium carbonate and talc at 10 minutes time.

The individual values *(y)* of analysis of calcium carbonate for three samples are 0.1055, 0.1055, and 0.1059 (in grams).

Solution:

At 10 minutes, time of blending, the data are processed as follows.

Samples	y values	$(y-\bar{y})$	$(y-\bar{y})^2$
1	0.1055	- 0.0001	1.0×10^4
2	0.1055	- 0.0001	1.0×10^{-8}
3	0.1059	0.0003	9.0×10^{-8}
Average, $\bar{y}$ =0.1056		$\Sigma (y-\bar{y})^2$ =	11.0×10^{-8}

Substituting the data in equation (15.1) gives

$$M_{10} = \sqrt{\frac{\Sigma(y-\bar{y})^2}{n(1-\bar{y})\bar{y}}} = \sqrt{\frac{11 \times 10^{-8}}{3(1-0.1056)0.1056}} = \sqrt{\frac{11 \times 10^{-8}}{0.2833}} = 0.00019$$

Per cent relative standard deviation (RSD)

$$= \frac{\text{Standard deviation}}{\text{Average}} \times 100 \quad \text{............(15.2)}$$

$$\text{Standard deviation} = \sqrt{\frac{\Sigma(y-\bar{y})^2}{(n-1)}} = \sqrt{\frac{11 \times 10^{-8}}{3-1}}$$

$$= \sqrt{5.5 \times 10^{-8}} = 2.345 \times 10^{-4}$$

$$RSD = \frac{2.345 \times 10^{-4}}{0.1056} \times 100 = 0.00222 \times 100 = 0.222\%$$

Preparation and Standardization of Solutions

Preparation of oxalic acid solution IP:

About 0.63 g of oxalic acid (molecular mass is 63 g/mol) is weighed and transferred into a 100-ml volumetric flask. Water is slowly added and shaken to dissolve the substance. Sufficient water is added to make 100 ml. Exact normality is calculated.

Weight of oxalic acid added, w = ____ g

Normality of oxalic acid solution, N1 $= \dfrac{w \times 10}{63} =$ _____ N

Preparation of sodium hydroxide (0.1 N) solution IP:

Solutions of any normality, xN, may be prepared by dissolving 40x g of sodium hydroxide in water and diluting to 1,000 ml. About 0.4 g of sodium hydroxide is weighed and transferred into 100 ml volumetric flask. Water is slowly added with continuous stirring, while cooling the flask under running tap water. Sufficient water is added to make 100 ml. The solution is allowed to stand overnight and decanted the clear liquid into a bottle. This clear liquid is used.

Standardization of sodium hydroxide (0.1 N) solution IP:

Ten ml of standardized oxalic acid solution is pipetted into conical flask. A drop of phenolphthalein indicator solution is added. The solution is titrated against sodium hydroxide solution placed in burette. Then, exact normality is calculated.

Burette: Sodium hydroxide solution

Conical flask: 10 ml oxalic acid solution Indicator: Phenolphthalein indicator solution

End point: Colorless to pink

OBSERVATIONS AND CALCULATIONS

Table 15.1: Titration Data for Estimation of Calcium Carbonate in the Blended Samples

Sampling time	Sample number	Volume of NaOH consumed	
		Initial volume, ml	Final volume, ml
(1)	(2)	(3)	(4)
At 10 min	1A		
	1B		
	1C		
At 20 min	2A		
	2B		
	2C		
At 30 min	3A		
	3B		
	3C		

~ 117 ~

Volume of NaOH consumed, (3) - (4), ml	Volume of HCl reacted with $CaCO_3$, ml (3) - (5) equivalent of HCl	Weight of $CaCO_3$, (6) x d, y	$(y-\bar{y})^2$
(5)	(6)	(7)	(8)
	Average, $\bar{y}$ =		$\sum (y-\bar{y})^2$ =
	Average, $\bar{y}$ =		$\sum (y-\bar{y})^2$ =
	Average, $\bar{y}$ =		$\sum (y-\bar{y})^2$ =

Burette readings	I	II	II
Initial reading, ml			
Final reading, ml			
Volume used, ml			

Section-IX   Expt-15: Mixing Index-Calcium carbonate and Talc

Average volume, $V_2 =$ ml

Normality of oxalic acid solution, $N_1 =$

Volume of oxalic acid solution taken, $V_1 = 10$ ml Volume of sodium hydroxide solution consumed, $V_2 =$

Normality of sodium hydroxide solution, $N_2 = \dfrac{N_1 V_1}{V_2}$

Preparation of hydrochloric acid (0.1 N) solution IP:

Solutions of any normality, x N, may be prepared by diluting 85x ml of hydrochloric acid to 1,000 ml with water. 250 ml of distilled water is taken into a 500-ml volumetric flask. 4.25 ml of concentrated hydrochloric acid is slowly added with continuous shaking. The flask is cooled under tap water. Distilled water is added to make the volume (500 ml) up to the mark.

Standardization of hydrochloric acid (0.1 N) solution IP:

Ten ml of hydrochloric acid solution is pipetted into a conical flask. A drop of phenolphthalein indicator solution is added. The solution is titrated against standardized sodium hydroxide solution placed in burette. Then exact normality is calculated.

Burette: Standardized sodium hydroxide solution

Conical flask: 10 ml hydrochloric acid solution

Indicator: Phenolphthalein

End point: Colorless to pink

Burette readings	I	II	II
Initial reading, ml			
Final reading, ml			
Volume used, ml			

Average volume, V_3 = _____ ml

Normality of sodium hydroxide solution, N_2 = _____ N

Volume of sodium hydroxide solution consumed, V_2 = 10 ml

Volume of Hydrochloric Acid solution taken, V_4 = 10 ml

Normality of hydrochloric acid solution, $N_3 = \dfrac{N_2 V_2}{V_4}$ = _____ N

Determination of conversion factor:

Accurately weighed 100 mg of calcium carbonate is placed in a conical flask (250 ml). 30 ml of hydrochloric acid solution (N_3 = N) is added. The contents are thoroughly shaken to ensure complete reaction. The unreacted hydrochloric acid is titrated against standard sodium hydroxide solution (N_2 = N). Conversion factor is calculated.

It is calculated with respect to calcium carbonate only, since talc is an inert material.

Burette: Standardized sodium hydroxide solution

Conical flask: 100 mg calcium carbonate + 30 ml standardized hydrochloric acid solution

Indicator: Phenolphthalein indicator solution

End point: Colorless to pink

Section-IX   Expt-15: Mixing Index-Calcium carbonate and Talc

Burette readings	I	II	II
Initial reading, ml			
Final reading, ml			
Volume used, ml			

Average volume, x = _____ ml

The volume of sodium hydroxide solution consumed, x =   ml

A mixture of 100 mg of $CaCO_3$ and 30 ml of (N_3 = _____N) HCl consumes x ml of (N_2 =_____N) NaOH solution. Unreacted HCl (N_3 =_____ N) in the mixture reacted with x ml of sodium hydroxide solution.

Normality of sodium hydroxide solution = N_2 = _____N

Volume of sodium hydroxide solution = x = _____ml

Normality of hydrochloric acid solution = N_3 = _____N

Equivalent volume of hydrochloric acid solution unreacted = $\dfrac{N_2.x}{N_3}$

= _____ ml *(e)*

(30.0 — e) ml of HCl (N_3 =_____N) reacts with 100 mg of $CaCO_3$

1 ml of HCl = 100 x 1 / (30.0 — e) *(c)* mg of calcium

= c/1000 = _____ *(d)* g of calcium carbonate

QUESTION BANK

1. Explain the principle involved in mixing of solids with a suitable example.
2. Name the different steps involved in solid-solid mixing.
3. Enumerate the applications of solids mixing.
4. Name a few equipment used for solids mixing.
5. How do you express the mixing of solids? Give an equation and explain the terms.
6. Describe the process of solid-solid mixing.

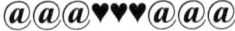

SECTION X
CRYSTALLIZATION

Expt-16: Effect of Various Factors on The Nature of Crystal Growth of Supersaturated Solutions by Different Methods.

AIM:

To observe the effects of various factors on the nature of crystal growth of a supersaturated solution by different methods

REQUIREMENTS:

Beakers, Any salt of potassium (KNO_3 or KCl), Glycerin, Urea, NaOH and water

PRINCIPLE:

Crystallization is a Unit operation, in which a solid is formed in its pure form from a homogeneous phase of solid either in liquid phase or in a vapour phase.

Crystallization mainly depends on *three (3)* conditions,

       1. A state of super saturation

       2. Formation of nuclei

       3. Growth of crystals

Depending on the condition of crystallization, it is possible to control or modify the nature of crystals obtained. The habit or shape of crystal form is highly depending on impurities in solution, pH, rate of cooling and solvent used.

Crystallization is mainly achieved by "super saturation". A super saturated solution can be obtained by different methods.
1. Super saturation by cooling method
2. Super saturation by evaporation
3. Super saturation by adiabatic evaporation (Cooling Evaporation)
4. Super saturation by salting out effect

If the solubility of a solvent depends on temperature i.e., if the solubility increases with an increase in temperature, super saturation can be brought about by cooling, leading to crystallization.

Adiabatic cooling plus evaporation are used for large-scale production.

In salting out method, addition of third substance reduces the solubility of solute up to the point where it crystallizes out.

PROCEDURE:

Preparation of super saturated solution:

Super saturated solution is one that contains more of the dissolved solute than it would normally contain at a definite temperature where the un-dissolved solute present.

Section-X — Expt-16: Effect of Factors on Crystal Growth

Prepare a saturated solution of a given salt by adding excess amount of salt in water (more than the solubility point), and decant the solution. Then collect the supernatant liquid and proceed for further steps.

Crystallization by Cooling:

Saturated solution of salt is taken at room temperature and divides into two portions in equal proportions and keeps in an ice bath. One of the containers is kept constantly without any shaking (disturbance) and the other is shaken continuously, till the growth of crystals observed in both containers. Note down the time and crystal shape, nature of the crystals observed microscopically.

Salting-Out Method:

Saturated solutions of salt is taken at room temperature and divides into three portions in equal proportions and add glycerin in one of the three portions, urea in one of the remaining two portions, NaOH in last portion of the remaining, and keep the containers aside for some time to form crystals. Then observe the crystal growth, and note down the time, shape of the crystals.

Take saturated solution and add glycerin with agitation and observe the growth of crystals, and determine the nature of the crystal growth under microscopically.

OBSERVATION:

Method of Crystallization	Time	Nature / Shape
Cooling without agitation		
Cooling with agitation		
Crystal form with Urea		
Crystal form with NaOH		
Crystal form with Glycerine		
Crystal form with Glycerine with agitation / stirring		

REPORT:

QUESTION BANK

1. Explain the theory of crystallization.
2. Define a) crystal; b) Crystal lattice; c) Crystal habit.
3. Enumerate different types of crystals.
4. Describe different methods by which super-saturation can be brought about.

Expt-17: Determination of Crystallization by Shock Cooling

AIM:

To study the crystallization behaviour of potassium nitrate and copper sulphate.

THEORY

Crystallization is the spontaneous arrangement of the particles (molecules, atoms, or ions) into a repetitive orderly array, i.e., regular geometric pattern. Crystals are commonly obtained from liquid state. The formation of crystals from solution involves 3 steps.

        1. Super saturation

        2. Nuclei formation

        3. Crystal growth

(1) Super saturation: When a solubility of a compound in a solvent exceeds the saturation solubility, the solution becomes supersaturated and the dissolved component may precipitate or crystallize. Supersaturation can be achieved by the following ways:

1. Evaporation of solvent from the solution.

2. Cooling of the solution, if the solute has positive heat of solution.
3. Formation of a new solute as a result of chemical reaction.
4. Addition of substance that is more soluble in solvent than the solid.

The rate of separation, particle size, uniformity, and distribution of crystals depend on nucleation and growth of nuclei.

(2) Nucleation: Nucleation refers to the birth of very small bodies of a new phase within a homogeneous supersaturated liquid phase.

Nucleation is a consequence of rapid local fluctuations at the molecular level when molecules, ions, or atoms are in random motion in any small volume. Initially several molecules, ions, or atoms associate to form clusters. These are loose aggregates, which usually disappear quickly.

The initially formed crystals are of molecular size and are termed as *nuclei*.

Several methods are available for nucleation. These are given below:

1. In a crystallizer, soft and weak crystals on impact with moving parts can break into fragments, which act as nuclei.

2. Small crystals which are formed in previous process are added to act as nuclei.
3. In a supersaturated solution or under poor mixing, needle like structures are observed at the ends of crystals. These structures grow faster than the sides of crystals, leading to form crystals of poor quality.

(3) Crystal growth:

Crystal growth is a diffusion process and surface phenomenon. From solution, solute molecules or ions reach the face of crystals by diffusion. On reaching the surface, the molecules or ions must be accepted by crystals and organized into space lattice. This phenomenon continues at the surface at a finite rate. Neither the diffusion nor the interfacial step will proceed unless, the solution is supersaturated.

In this experiment, supersaturation by shock cooling technique is used to crystallize potassium nitrate from the saturated solution. Crystallization can be studied in a similar manner using copper sulphate, salicylic acid, acetanilide, and sodium chloride. However, rate of crystallization is relatively less in sodium chloride and copper sulphate than in potassium nitrate.

PRINCIPLE

Potassium nitrate crystals can be obtained using shock cooling technique. The solid (solute) is added to a solvent continuously until the solid is dissolved. Such a solution is called as saturated solution. The rate of dissolution process is enhanced by increasing the temperature and agitation. When some solid remained undissolved, then such a solution is called as super saturated solution. When the temperature of supersaturated solution is decreased rapidly (shock cooling), the solubility of solute decreases. As a result, the dissolved solid gets crystallized, through the processes of nucleation and crystal growth. The extent of crystallization depends on the time of contact in low temperature. The crystals are collected by filtration and weighed. Yield is expressed as per cent weight of crystals obtained. A graph is plotted taking time versus per cent weight of crystals as shown in **Figure**.

REQUIREMENTS

Beaker, 250 ml; Potassium nitrate; Weighing balance; Ice bath; Water bath; Stop watch; Test tubes, 10 ml; Measuring cylinder, 100 ml; Hair dryer; Microscope; (or magnifying lens); Funnel; Filter paper.

PROCEDURE

1. 25 grams of potassium nitrate is accurately weighed (W_1 g).
2. Hundred ml water is transferred into 250 ml beaker.
3. Beaker containing water is placed in constant temperature water bath maintained at 50°C.

4. Potassium nitrate is added into the water little by little, the solution is stirred with glass rod to dissolve the solute.
5. This process is continued until saturated solution (with little excess crystals) is formed.

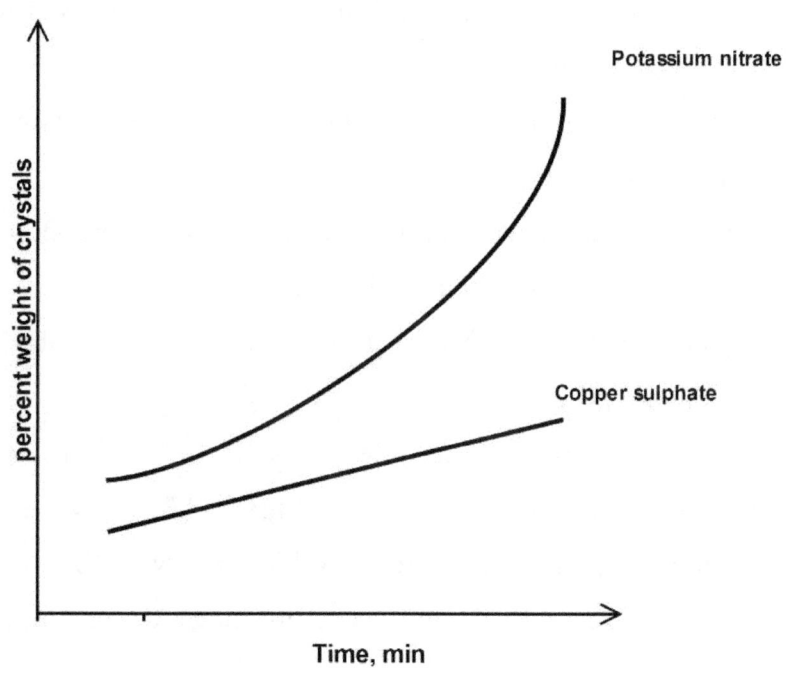

Figure 17.1: Crystallization curves of potassium nitrate and copper sulphate

6. Weight of potassium nitrate remained is weighed (W_2 g). Difference in the weights W g (W_1-W_2) gives weight of potassium nitrate added into 100 ml water.

7. From this, 10 ml quantities of saturated solution are transferred into 9 test tubes.
8. All the test tubes are placed in an ice bath at once. Temperature of the solution decreases suddenly due to shock cooling forming supersaturated solution (Rate of cooling can be maintained constant by keeping the test tubes either in constant temperature water-bath maintained at 20°C or in refrigerator). Nucleation and crystal growth takes place.
9. After 10 minutes, the solution of first test tube is filtered to collect crystals.
10. This is repeated after every 10 minutes thereafter using the solutions of other test tubes.
11. All the crystals collected on the filter paper separately are subjected to drying using hair dryer.
12. eights of each sample of crystals are recorded in **Table-17.1**, and data is processed.
13. A graph is plotted taking time on x-axis and per cent weight of crystals on y-axis as shown in **Figure-17.1.** Crystal habit of potassium nitrate, before and after crystallization, is studied under microscope (or using magnifying lens) and reported.

Section-X   Expt-17: Crystallization-Shock Cooling

OBSERVATIONS AND CALCULATIONS:

Table 17.1: Data for the Crystallization of Potassium Nitrate

Test tube No.	Time in min	Weight of crystals formed, g (b)	Percentage weight of crystals b/a x 100
1	10		
2	20		
3	30		
4	40		
5	50		
6	60		
7	70		
8	80		
9	90		

a = Weight of Potassium Nitrate present in 10 ml of water, g

	Before Crystallization	After Crystallization
Crystal habit of Potassium Nitrate		

REPORT

Per cent weight of potassium nitrate crystals formed in 90 min =

QUESTION BANK

1. What are the pharmaceutical applications of crystallization?
2. Describe the principle involved in the crystallization with a suitable example.
3. List the methods used for nucleation in the crystallization process.
4. Explain the process of crystal growth in the crystallization process.

DEFINITIONS

DRYING

Drying: Drying is defined as the removal of small amounts of water or other liquid from a material by the application of heat.

Bound water: Bound water is the minimum water held by the material that exerts an equilibrium vapour pressure less than the pure water at the same temperature.

Unbound water: unbound water is the amount of water held by the material that exerts an equilibrium vapour presser equal to that of pure water at the same temperature.

Equilibrium moisture content (EMC): *It* is the amount of water present in the solid that exerts a vapour pressure equal to the vapour pressure of the atmosphere surrounding it.

Hygroscopic Substances: Substances containing bound water are often called hygroscopic substances.

Non-hygroscopic Substances: Substances containing unbound water are often called non-hygroscopic substances.

Desorption: When air is continuously passed over the solid containing moisture more than EMC, then solid losses water continuously till EMC is reached. This phenomenon is known as desorption.

Sorption: When air is continuously passed over the solid containing moisture less than EMC, then solid adsorb water continuously till EMC is reached. This phenomenon is known as sorption.

Free moisture content (FMC): Free moisture content (FMC) is the amount of water that is free to evaporate from the solid surface.

Drying rate: The ratio of weight of water (kg) in sample by time into weight of the dry solid.

% Loss on drying: The % ratio of mass of water in sample (kg) by total mass of the wet sample (kg).

% Moisture Content (MC): The % ratio of mass of water in sample (kg) by mass of the dry sample (kg).

Drying rate curve: *A graph is plotted between FMC on X-axis and drying rate on Y-axis, the curve so obtained is called drying rate curve.*

Critical Moisture Content: *The rate of diffusion is equal to the rate of evaporation. The moisture content at the end of constant rate is referred to as the critical moisture content.*

Definitions

Eutectic Point: *The pressure and temperature at which the frozen solid vaporizes without conversion to a liquid is referred to as the eutectic point.*

Mier's Theory: *Under ideal conditions of crystallization nucleus formation starts at super solubility curve and crystal growth begins.*

CRYSTALLIZATION

Crystallization: *crystallization is the spontaneous arrangement of the particles into a repetitive orderly array i.e., regular geometric patterns.*

Sublimation: *Crystallization can take place directly from vapour of a substance, ex: Solid camphor from camphor vapour, solid iodine from iodine vapour such process is known as sublimation.*

Crystal: *A crystal can be defined as a solid particle, which is formed by the solidification process in which structural units are arranged, by a fixed geometric pattern or lattice.*

Crystal lattice: *It is defined as an orderly internal arrangement of particles in three-dimensional spaces.*

Space lattice: *The three-dimensional arrangement of particles in a crystal is also known as space lattice.*

Unit cell: *The smallest geometric portion, which repeats to build up the whole crystal, is called a Unit cell.*

Faces: *A crystal is bounded by plane surfaces called faces.*

Axial Angle: *In the crystal, the angle between the two perpendiculars to the intersecting faces is termed as the axial angle.*

Axial Length: *Axial length can be defined as the distance between the centers of two atoms.*

Crystal system (or) forms: *A finite number of symmetrical arrangements are possible for a crystal lattice and these may be termed as crystal forms or systems.*

Crystal Habit: *The term crystal habit is used to denote the relative development of the different types of faces and not to the shape of the resulting crystals.*

Crystalline Solids: Crystals that have definite shape and an orderly arrangement of units of incompressible is called as crystalline solids.

Amorphous Solids: Amorphous solid do not have specific shape and their structural units are arranged randomly in the solid.

Polymorphs: Certain drugs can exist in more than one crystalline form. Such a phenomenon is known as polymorphism.

Drug Hydrates: Some drugs have greater tendency to associate with water. The resulting substance is referred to as drug hydrates.

Definitions

Pseudomorphs : Certain drugs have greater tendency to associate with solvents to produce crystalline forms of solvates. These solvates are also known as pseudomorphs.

Isomorphism: When two or more substances possess the same crystalline form, the crystals of one such substance can be grown in the saturated solution of the other. This phenomenon is known as isomorph ism.

Nucleation: Nucleation refers to the birth of very small bodies of a new phase within a homogenous supersaturated liquid phase.

Crystal Growth: Crystal growth is a diffusion process and surface phenomenon, in which solute molecules or ions reach the faces of a crystal by diffusion, and organized into space lattice.

Meta-stable state: The region enclosed between the two curves called normal solubility curve AB and super solubility curve FG is referred as meta-stable state.

Solubility curve: The graph drawn by taking temperature on X-axis and solubility on Y-axis gives the solubility curve.

Caking of crystals: Caking can be defined as the process of formation of clumps or cakes when crystals are improperly stored.

Critical Humidity: Critical humidity is the humidity above which crystals absorb moisture and below which they do not absorb moisture.

Cubic: Three equal axes at right angle to each other.

Tetragonal: Three axis all right angles, one longer than the other two.

Orthorhombic: Three axes all at right angle, but all of different lengths.

Hexagonal: Three equal axes in one plane at 60° to each other, one at right angle to this plane but not necessarily the same length as the other.

Monoclinic: Two axes at right angles in one plane, and a third axis at some odd angle to this plane.

Triclinic: Three axes at odd angles to each other.

DISTILLATION

Distillation: Distillation is defined as the separation of the components of a liquid mixture by a process involving vaporization and subsequent condensation at another place.

Simple Distillation: It is a process of converting a single constituent from a liquid (mixture) into its vapour transferring the vapour to another place & recovering the liquid by condensing the vapour, usually by allowing it to come in contact with cold surface. This is also known as **Differential distillation.**

Flash Distillation: It is defined as a process in which the entire liquid mixture is suddenly vapourized (flash) by passing the feed from a high-pressure zone to a low pressure. It is also known as **Equilibrium distillation.**

Fractional distillation: It is a process in which vapourization of liquid mixture gives rise to a mixture of constituents from which the desired one is separated in pure form. This is also known as **Rectification.**

Reflux ratio: It is the quotient of the amount of liquid returning through the column to the amount collected into the receiver during the same interval of time.

Azeotropic Distillation: It is a method in which azeotropic mixture is broken by the addition of a third substance, which forms a new azeotrope with one of the components.

Extractive Distillation: It is a distillation method in which the third substance added to azeotropic mixture is relatively non-volatile liquid compared to the components to be separated.

Distillation Under Reduced Pressure: It is defined as distillation process in which the liquid is distilled at a temperature lower than its boiling point by the application of vacuum.

Steam Distillation: It is a method of distillation carried with the aid of steam and is used for the separation of high boiling substances from nonvolatile impurities.

Molecular Distillation: It is defined as a distillation process in which each molecule in the vapour phase travels mean free path and it's condensed individually without intermolecular collisions on application of vacuum.

Mean free path: It is defined as the average distance through which a molecule can move without coming into collisions with another.

Destructive Distillation: It is a distillation method in which the distillate is decomposition products of the constituents of the organic matter burnt in the absence of air. This process is also known as **Dry distillation.**

Distilland: The feed liquid is known as Distilland.
Condensate: The condensed liquid is known as condensate.

Binary mixture of liquids: When two liquids are mixed together, they may be miscible with each other in all proportions. Such miscible liquids are known as binary mixture of liquid.

Raoult's Law: Raoult's law stated that the partial vapour pressure of each volatile constituent is equal to the vapour pressure of the pure constituent multiplied by its mole fraction in the solution at a given temperature.

Definitions

Ideal solution: Ideal solution is defined, as the one in which there is no change in the properties of the components other than dilution, when they are mixed to form a solution.

Perfect solution: Raoult's law is obeyed by only a few solutions of liquid in liquids. These solutions are know\ n as perfect solutions.

Real solution: Real solution is defined as the one, which show varying degrees of deviation from Raoult's law.

Dalton's law: Dalton's law of partial vapour pressure states that the total pressure exerts by a mixture of ideal gases may be considered as sum of the partial vapour pressure exerted by each gas, if alone were present and occupied the total volume.

Positive deviation: The vapour pressure is greater than the sum of the partial pressures of the individual components. Such systems are said to exhibit positive deviation from raoult's law.

Negative deviation: The vapour pressure is lower than the sum of the partial pressures of the individual components. Such systems are said to exhibit negative deviation from raoult's law.

Volatility: The volatility of any substance in a solution is defined as the equilibrium partial pressure of the substance in the vapour phase divided by the mole fraction of the substance in the solution.

Relative volatility: Relative volatility is defined as a ratio of volatility of two components (component A to the volatility of component B).

Azeotrope: Many liquid mixtures cannot be separated completely into pure components by simple distillation, because the volatilities of the components are equal. Such a mixture is known as azeotrope.

Azeotropic solution: Azeotropic solution is a solution, which distils unchanged at a constant temperature (Constant boiling mixtures).

Azeotropic mixture: The system that exhibits a maximum value in the boiling point composition such a system is known as azeotropic mixture with a minimum vapour pressure or maximum boiling point.

HUMIDITY AND AIRCONDITION

Humidity: The pounds of water vapour carried by one pound of dry air under any given set of conditions is known as Humidity.

Saturated air: The air in which the water vapour is in equilibrium with liquid water at the given conditions of temperature and pressure is called saturated air.

Saturated Humidity: The water vapour, which is present in the saturated air, is called saturated humidity.

Definitions

Percentage Humidity: % humidity is the ratio of weight of water vapour carried by one pound of dry air at any temperature and pressure to the weight of water one pound of dry air could carry if saturated at same temperature and pressure, and expressing in the result on a percentage basis.

% Relative Humidity: It is the ratio of the partial pressure of water vapour in the air-water vapour mixture to the partial pressure of water vapour at saturation (Liquid water).

Humid Heat: Humid heat is a number of Btu necessary to raise the temperature of one pound of dry air plus whatever water vapour it may carry by one °F.

Enthalpy: Enthalpy of air-water vapour mixture is the enthalpy of one pound of dry air plus the enthalpy of accompanying water vapour.

Humid Volume: Humid volume is the volume in Cu. ft. occupied by one pound of dry air and its accompanying water vapour.

Saturated Volume: It is the volume in Cu. ft of one pound of dry air plus that of the water vapour necessary to saturate it.

Dew Point: It is the temperature to which a mixture of air and water vapour must be cooled in order to become saturate. It is also known as Saturation Temperature.

Dry bulb Temperature: It is a temperature of moist air, when it is measured at rest by any instrument, which is not effected by the moisture content of air or by radiation.

Wet bulb Temperature: It is the dynamic equilibrium temperature attained by a water surface when exposed to air under adiabatic conditions.

Adiabatic Saturation Temperature: When water is sprayed into a stream of gas, equilibrium is reached between gas and water. Then the temperature of gas is called adiabatic saturation temperature.

Humidity Chart: A convenient diagram, which shows the properties of mixtures of a permanent gas and a condensable vapour is called humidity chart.

Air Conditioning: It is a process of treating air, so as to control simultaneously its temperature, humidity, cleanliness and distribution to meet the requirements of the conditioned space.

Humidification: It is a Unit operation, which involves a transfer of liquid water into water vapour.

Dehumidification: The process in which the moisture is decreased (Transfer of vapour to liquid state) in the air is known as dehumidification.

Latent heat of Vapourization : It is defined as the quantity of heat required to convert a unit mass of the liquid at its boiling point from the liquid to the vapour state without a change in temperature.

FLOW OF HEAT

Conduction: When heat flow in a body by the transfer of momentum of individual atoms or molecules without mixing, such process is known as conduction.

Convection: When heat is achieved by actual mixing of warmer portion with cooler portion of same material, this process is known as convection.

Radiation: When the heat flows through space by means of electromagnetic waves is known as radiation.

Forced convection: Mixing of fluid may be obtained by the use of a stirrer or agitator or pumping the fluid for re-circulation. Such a process in heat transfer is designated as forced convection.

Natural convection: When a fluid is heated, the current setup may cause mixing of fluid. Such a heat transfer process is known as natural convection.

Film coefficient: Film coefficient is the quantity of heat flowing through unit area of the filth for unit drop in temperature.

Parallel heat flow: When the hot fluid and the cold fluid enter the apparatus from the same end, the flow is parallel to each other. This arrangement is known as parallel flow.

Counter-current heat flow: When the hot fluid is passed through one end of the apparatus while cold fluid is passed through the other end. fluids pass and by pass each other in the opposite directions. This arrangement is known as counter-current or counter flow.

Thermal radiation: Heat transfer by radiation is known as thermal radiation.

Black body: Black body is defined as a body that radiates maximum possible amount of energy at a given temperature.

Grey body: Grey body is defined as a body whose absorptivity is constant at all wavelengths of radiation, at a given temperature.

Emissivity: The energy emitted by actual body to the energy emitted black body is known as emissivity.

Heat exchangers: Heat exchangers are the devices used for transferring, heat from one fluid (hot gas or stream) to another fluid (liquid) through a metal wall.

Heat interchangers: Heat interchangers are the devices used for transferring heat from one liquid to another or from one gas to another gas through a metal wall.

EVAPORATION

Evaporation: Evaporation is a process of vaporizing large quantities of volatile liquid to get a concentrated product. (Or) The process of removal of solvent from the solution by boiling the liquid in a suitable vessel, and withdrawing the vapour, leaving a concentrated liquid residue in the vessel, is called evaporation.

Entrainment: The phenomenon in which finely divided liquid droplets are carried along with the stream of vapour is called entrainment.

Foam: Foam is the formation of a stable blanket of bubbles that lies on the surface of boiling milk (boiling liquids).

Calandria: Calandria is a steam compartment, which consists of a number of tubes fitted in a vessel and is included in the evaporator.

SIZE REDUCTION & SIZE SEPARATION

Size reduction: Size reduction is a process of reducing large solid unit masses into small unit masses, coarse particles or fine particles. It is also termed as comminution or diminution or pulverization.

Cutting: Cutting is a means of tearing the material by a sharp blade.

Compression: Compression is a means by which the material is crushed between rollers by the application of pressure.

Attrition: Attrition involves breaking down of the material by rubbing action between two surfaces.

Impact: It involves the operation of splitting the material apart, when a lump of material strikes against the rotating hammers.

Size separation: Size separation is a unit operation that involves the separation of a mixture of various sizes of particles into two or more portions by means of screening surfaces. It also known as sieving / sifting / classifying / screening.

Coarse powder: A powder, all the particles of which pass through a sieve with nominal mesh aperture of 1.7 mm (No. 10 sieve) and not more than 40% through a sieve with nominal mesh aperture of 355 gm. (No. 44 sieve) is called coarse powder.

Sieve number: Sieve number indicates the number of meshes per linear length of 0.0254 m (one inch).

Blending: It means to mix smoothly and inseparably together.

Centrifugation: *It* is a unit operation employed for separating the constituents present in dispersion with the aid of centrifugal force.

Actual Screen: It is the one that does not give perfect separation about the cut diameter.

MIXING

Mixing: Mixing is defined as a process that tends to result in a randomization of dissimilar particles with in a system

Connective mixing: It is achieved by the inversion of the powder bed using blades or paddles or screw element.

Shear mixing: In this type, the forces of attraction are broken down so that each particle moves on its own between regions of different composition and parallel to their surfaces.

Diffusive mixing: It involves the random motion of particles within the powder bed there by particles change their positions relative to one another.

Agitation: Agitation refers to the induced motion of a material in a specified way, usually in a circulatory pattern inside a container.

Bulk Transport: Bulk transport is defined as the movement of a large portion of a material from one location to another location in a given system.

Turbulent mixing: Turbulent mixing is defined as mixing due to turbulent flow, which results in random fluctuation of the fluid velocity at any given point within the system.

Laminar mixing: Laminar mixing is the mixing of two dissimilar liquids through laminar flow, i.e. the applied shear stretches the interface between them.

Molecular Diffusion: Molecular diffusion is the mixing at molecular level in which molecules diffuse due to thermal motion.

Pitch: Pitch is defined as the distance the impeller would move through the fluid per revolution, if slippage does not occur.

FILTRATION

Filtration: Filtration may be defined as a process of separation of solids from a fluid by passing the same through a porous medium that retains the solids, but allows the fluid to pass though.

Slurry: The suspension to be filtered is known as slurry.

Filter medium: The porous medium used to retain the solids is known as filter medium.

Filter cake: The accumulated solids on the filter are referred to as filter cake.

Filtrate: The clear liquid passing through the filter is filtrate.

Surface Filtration: It is a screening action by which pores or holes of the medium prevent the passage of solids. It is also known as screen filtration.

Depth Filtration: In this process, slurry penetrates to a point where the diameter of solid particles is greater than that of the void or channel.

Cake Filtration: A filter consists of a coarse woven cloth through which a concentrated suspension of rigid particles is passed, so that they bridge the holes and form a bed.

Filter Aid: It forms a surface deposit, which screens out the solids and also prevents plugging of the supporting filter medium.

Clarification: It is the process of separation of low concentration of solids (<1% w/v) from liquid.

VIVA QUESTIONS

I. Radiation Constant of Iron Cylinder

II. Radiation Constant of Brass Cylinder

III. Radiation Constant of Copper Cylinder

IV. Painted Glass

V. Unpainted Glass

1. What do you mean by radiation constant?
2. What do you mean by Conduction, Convection & Radiation?
3. What is Stephan Boltzman constant?
4. What is black body?
5. Why do you prefer Iron, Brass & Copper cylinders for determining Radiation Constant?
6. What is your intention to do this experiment?
7. How the temperature will influence on Radiation Constant?
8. What are incandescent solids?
9. In how many ways heat can be transferred to the metal walls?
10. What are the Pharmaceutical applications of Radiation Constant?

VI. Size Reduction & Seperation

1. What are the synonyms for size reduction?
2. Why size reduction is extensively used in Pharmaceutical operations?
3. What are the mechanisms involved in size reduction?
4. What are the applications of size reduction?
5. What are the objectives of size reduction?
6. What is the principle involved in ball mill?
7. Why do you get different sizes of particles?
8. Why do you prefer same size of Balls?

VII. Flow of Fluids

1. What is streamline flovv & turbulent flow?
2. What do you mean by Reynolds Number?
3. What is critical velocity?
4. What are the factors that affect the fluid flow?
5. What are the limitations of Reynolds Number?
6. What is the significance of Reynolds Number?
7. How does viscosity of liquid, diameter & length of the pipe affect the friction?
8. In which flow Eddies are formed?

VIII. Drying

1. What is the mechanism involved in Drying operation?
2. What are the different stages of drying?
3. What is critical moisture content?
4. What do you mean by first falling period?

5. What are the factors that affect the rate of Drying?
6. What is the importance of Drying?
7. What are the Pharmaceutical applications of drying?
8. What is equilibrium moisture content?

IX. Particle Size Analysis

1. What are the different types of powders?
2. What is the type of arrangement of sieves during sieve analysis?
3. What do mean by tailing?
4. What are fines & tails?
5. What are least & maximum size of particles Pharmaceutically?
6. Why different sizes of particles used in preparation of Tablets?
7. In which area of pharmaceutical operations sieves analysis is used?
8. What are the specifications of standard sieves?

X. FILTRATION

1. What is filter aid & give some examples?
2. What do you mean by filtration?
3. What are the factors affecting the rate of filtration?
4. How does the particle size affect the rate of filtration?
5. What is the equation that governs the effect of particle size on rate of filtration?
6. In how many ways filter aids can be used?
7. What are the applications of filtration in Industrial Pharmacy?

Viva Questions

8. What are the different types of Filtration mechanisms?

XI. Humidity

1. What is Humidity?
2. What is Dry bulb & Wet bulb temperatures?
3. What is adiabatic temperature?
4. What are adiabatic cooling lines?
5. What relative Humidity?
6. What do you mean by Dew point?
7. What is the use of Humidity chart?
8. What are the different methods to find Humidity?

XII. Crystallization

1. What are the operations involved in crystallization'?
2. What are the different ways to achieve super saturation?
3. What is salting out method?
4. What do you mean by adiabatic evaporation?
5. How the nuclei will form?
6. What do you mean the term Crystal growth?
7. What are the factors that affect the crystallization?
8. What is the effect of pH on crystallization?
9. What is solubility?
10. What effect of temperature on solubility?

XIII. Distillation

1. What are the applications of distillation in Pharmacy?
2. What do you mean by vapour pressure?

3. What do you mean by boiling point?
4. What is relative volatility?
5. Classify the types of distillations?
6. What is steam distillation?
7. What do you mean Azeotrope (Entrainers)?
8. What are the applications of Azeotropic distillation?
9. How can prepare the aromatic water?
10. What are different types of Azeotropic mixtures & give examples?
11. What is use of boiling point diagram?
12. What are colligative properties?

XIV. Stokes Law

1. What is stokes law?
2. What are the factors affecting the stokes law
3. What are the limitations of stokes law
4. Name some Pharmaceutical dosage forms where stokes law is applicable?
5. What do you mean by Terminal settle velocity?
6. What are the applications of stokes law?
7. What is viscosity?
8. What is the viscosity of glycerin?

XV. Centrifugation

1. What is Centrifugation?
2. What do you mean by Centrifugal force?
3. What do you mean by driving force?

4. What are the different types of Centrifuges?

5. What are the factors that affect the Centrifuges?

6. What are suspending agents & give examples?

XVI. Extraction

1. What is maceration?
2. What is percolation?
3. What do you mean by tinctures & galanicals?
4. Enumerate different methods of maceration?
5. Enumerate different methods of percolation?
6. What do you mean Menstruum?
7. What is marc?
8. What is digestion?
9. What is infusion?
10. What is decoction?
11. What is effect of temperature on extraction?

@@@♥♥@@@

BIBLIOGRAPHY

Introduction to chemical engineering, 7th Edition, by Walter L. Badger and Juliust T. Banchero.

Pharmaceutical Engineering principles and practices, 6th Edition, by C.V.S. Subrahmanyam,

Cooper and Gun's, Tutorial Pharmacy, 6th Edition, Edited by S.J. Carter.

Pharmaceutical Engineering, 2003 1st Edition, by K. Sambamurthy.

Unit operations of chemical engineering, 6th Edition, by M.C. Cabe, Smith, Harriott.

Pharmaceutical engineering practical manual (Unit Operations), Sudhakar Reddy P, Pharma Book Syndicate.

NOTES